Mindful Pause

A Self-Care Guide to
Resilience and Well-Being

Stop. Breathe. Think. Choose.

Mindful Pause

A Self-Care Guide to Resilience and Well-Being

Stop. Breathe. Think. Choose.

CAMI SMALLEY

Niche Pressworks
Indianapolis

MINDFUL PAUSE

ISBN   978-1-946533-70-8 paperback
        978-1-946533-91-3 ebook

The information in this book is not intended as a substitute for consultation with healthcare professionals. Each individual's health concerns should be evaluated by a qualified professional.

Grateful acknowledgement is made for permission to reprint the **"Heart Rhythm"** image, copyright HeartMath Institute, 1997.

For permission to reprint portions of this content or bulk purchases, contact the author, Cami Smalley:

Cami@GuidedResilience.com

Published by Niche Pressworks, Indianapolis, http://NichePressworks.com

The views of the author do not necessarily represent the views of the publisher.

Printed in the United States of America

I dedicate this book
to my husband and best friend, Steve.
Whenever I stop, breathe, think ...
I always choose you.

Acknowledgements

To my family and friends as well as the many teachers, coaches, and institutions whose presence in my life have formed, challenged, and inspired my personal practice of Mindful Pause, including: St. Catherine University, University of Northern Iowa, Wellcoaches, YogaFit, Rebecca McClean, and Jane Toerner. Additionally, the inspirations and work of the following guided my own resilience: St. Francis of Assisi, Richard Rohr, Jon Kabat-Zinn, Herbert Benson, Thomas Keating, Thich Nhat Hanh, Pema Chodron, and Cynthia Bourgeault.

To Regions Hospital in St. Paul, MN, for being a champion of my Guided Resilience wellness coaching and for supporting my resilience work with employees across the organization including environmental services, birth center, nursing education, coding, mental health occupational therapists, cardiology, and the emergency department to name a few. Additionally, my friends and colleagues in the Employee Health Department at Regions have been invaluable. Their energy and enthusiasm inspire me on a daily basis.

The following publishers and/or authors have generously given permission to reprint material from copyrighted works:

The **Heart Rhythm** image, copyright 1997 by HeartMath Institute.

Contents

THINK

CHOOSE

Introduction

Self-Care Crisis

*In order to change, we must be sick
and tired of being sick and tired.*

–Anonymous

The pace and intensity of life today are leaving people exhausted and disconnected from the self they once knew or aspired to be. The belief in happiness as a reward for hard work seems a false hope. People are fractured from overextending themselves in work, life, and relationships and often find themselves disillusioned and set on a course for a personal breakdown.

The incidence of burned-out professionals, exhausted caregivers, and overextended volunteers is on the rise. Survivors of chronic disease, workplace violence, career transitions, or wounded or broken relationships feel robbed of the "good life" they once knew.

Critical life events often prompt the need for support. Uncertainty can be scary and unfamiliar territory. But uncomfortable life moments are also opportunities for change and can lead to personal growth. It's easy to be consumed by frustration, overwhelm, disappointment, or loss, igniting a sense of hopelessness, confusion, or fatigue. Resilience is tested.

It's time to detour onto another path to pursue new skills, grow your confidence, and strengthen your resilience through tough times. This book provides support for the overstretched and dangerously driven who endlessly serve, undoubtedly suffer, and are ready to seek relief.

Remedy: Mindful Pause

The unexamined life is not worth living.

–Socrates

Life and culture are moving at casualty pace. People are hurried … harried … and hopelessly unaware of the risks of an "unexamined life."

This book is for those who are ready to live the power of pause. Mindful Pause guides you to stop, breathe, think, and choose to wake up to things that make life deeply meaningful and purposeful. That takes time. The wellness journey is NOT like fast food, photos in a flash, movies on demand, or Instagram.

It's no wonder many feel fractured and overwhelmed.

Many don't acknowledge self-care as a necessity for personal and professional health and well-being. And even those who do often lack the self-regulation skills to remedy the impact of demanding lives. With honest self-reflection and some easy to apply self-care skills, you can endure difficult times and come out more resilient on the other side.

In recent decades, mind-body disciplines and positive psychology coaching have demonstrated the necessity for wellness and self-care to support health and well-being. As a professional wellness coach, I invite you to pause in the busyness or upset of life. Take a moment to engage in a strategy that helps manage difficult emotions and skillfully aligns thoughts and actions with beliefs, strengths, and values to achieve personal and professional well-being.

It is good to have an end to journey toward;
but it is the journey that matters, in the end.

–Ursula K. Le Guin

A personal wellness journey is worth the work. You know dedication. You have applied your drive. And it's taken you to a cliff. Step away from the edge and look around. You deserve relief, and it is within your reach. You can generate and sustain the energy and outlook you need to live life to the fullest.

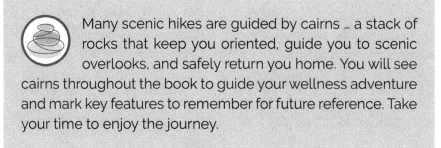

Many scenic hikes are guided by cairns … a stack of rocks that keep you oriented, guide you to scenic overlooks, and safely return you home. You will see cairns throughout the book to guide your wellness adventure and mark key features to remember for future reference. Take your time to enjoy the journey.

Avoid crisis and choose adventure. Anchoring your mind and heart to inner peace and tested wisdom generates the inspiration to pursue a new way of being. You will discover the courage, the means, and the confidence to navigate through (or sometimes around) bumps in the road. The seemingly impassable trenches teach you perseverance, and dead ends invite you to learn from your mistakes and change your route.

Wherever your journey begins, you can benefit from the personal growth that comes through your thoughtful engagement, conscious effort, and personal commitment to pause.

When you see this symbol throughout the book, I'm inviting you to pause for self-reflection, personal assessment, or an exercise. So, get out your journal. You will experience important moments along the way. Record them. There will be moments of insight that you'll want to savor.

The common barrier to personal growth? Time. But that excuse will not work anymore. The qualities of wisdom and peace are often significantly diminished, completely absent, overlooked, or exhausted when overwhelmed with stress. I invite you to prioritize self-care by taking time to work through this book.

> Those who think they don't have time for self-care will sooner or later have to make time for the demise of well-being.

Life's disruptions don't have to end in chaos, dis-ease, or despair. And the pace of life and work do not have to end in burnout. You can achieve and sustain inner peace and stability that supports good living.

It isn't enough to talk about peace. One must believe in it. And it isn't enough to believe in it. One must work at it.

–Eleanor Roosevelt

This book is divided into four parts, and the chapters walk you through the Mindful Pause process. Part I, Stop, addresses your personal need to stop and introduces what we mean by resilience. Part II, Breathe, gives more in-depth instruction on self-regulation. Part III, Think, explores two key areas of positive psychology coaching—values (or strengths) and positive emotions—as well as some nuggets of wisdom from my coaching practice. And Part IV, Choose, offers self-care practices that support the Mindful Pause process.

Difficult moments can be endured, observed, and masterfully transformed into a stronger version of you. Follow the cairns, and you will not regret this journey toward personal well-being.

Stop

*Tell me, what is it you plan to do
with your one wild and precious life?*

–Mary Oliver

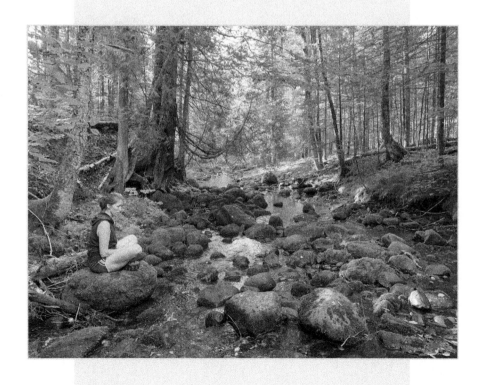

Chapter 1

Read the Signs ...

There's more to life than
increasing its speed.

–Gandhi

Stop signs are posted to alert drivers at hazardous or complex intersections. **How** you live (or drive) ... and **why** you stop are discussed in this chapter. Many are living at a pace that is unsustainable. They ignore warning signals, speed limits, and invitations to stop and enjoy the view. The increase in speed and complexity of life often intensifies without notice, especially if everyone around you is keeping a similar pace!

Because we do not rest, we sometimes lose our way. More than one client has pursued coaching because they "no longer recognize themselves." Their formerly happy, healthy self has been hijacked by the circumstances of their life. It's easy to become separated from the stillness from which wisdom grows. We miss the joy and peace born of mindful presence. Without pause, the inspiration of moments, people, and our environment elude us and leave us longing for something more ... when there is a whole lot of something right in front of us.

Sometimes stopping can be forced upon us. The forced stops may be necessitated by any number of life circumstances that leave you feeling depleted, confused, anxious, frustrated, dissatisfied, or off-track. Intentional stops interrupt the dangerous speeds that many have acclimated to in life.

Some pursue coaching for more resilience. But is more resilience really what people need? Sometimes. We will take a look at several determinants that impact your wellness lifestyle. You will assess your resilience and explore the mindset of self-care and your holistic well-being. We will also consider the common challenges of time and stress in daily life.

You are at an intersection moment of life. Examine your whole life … and you are likely to reveal a turn onto a more life-giving path. You have everything you need to navigate your journey with more ease than you thought possible.

Why Stop?

Think back to when you were in elementary school. What were you taught to do if your clothes catch on fire?

Stop, drop, and roll.

Have you ever had the occasion to use this remedy?

Fortunately, most of us have not. But most seem to be able to recall it quickly. It's catchy and easy to remember. This simplicity is applied to the steps that you can take to put out the *metaphorical fires* that come up in life. How often does that happen? For most of us, frequently.

Task loading, constant interruptions, career changes, traffic jams, demanding colleagues, difficult clients, patients, partners, or children. The list goes on.

So now that we're all grown up, we can remember four simple steps to put out the metaphorical fires that inflame our lives:

Stop. Breathe. Think. Choose.

These steps will remedy your self-care crisis.

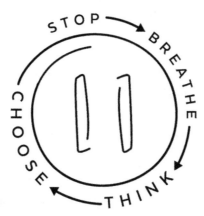

These simple steps guide you through a self-care process that transforms stress, challenge, or adversity by the mindful integration of body, mind, and spirit. The process focuses on connecting you back to yourself. It helps you remember and align with the inner qualities of peace and stability to empower choices that lead to optimal health and satisfaction in life, work, and relationships. Self-care helps you shift gears.

Clients often post these four simple words as a reminder for how to navigate difficult moments. I needed a reference for these steps, and the cue "Mindful Pause" was born. Sometimes the most simple words are enough to inspire profound change.

Accept this invitation to pause ... to douse the fire of stress in your life and to make room for vitality and growth. Unplug from the incessant pace of modern culture to align with your purpose and strengths, manage mood and energy with confidence, and seek growth and transformation. This is especially critical for those who feel separated from themselves by an exhaustive effort to work harder and achieve more, while simultaneously prioritizing and caring for others.

We need to STOP. But stopping to rest and practice self-care is so contradictory to our cultural addiction to work and productivity. This strong work ethic is producing a population that is literally sick and tired from the pursuit of the American dream. Consider these population statistics:

- Nearly half of Americans (45 percent) have been awake at night in the past month as one stress outcome.[1]

- Forty-two percent of adults say they are not doing enough or are unsure if they are doing enough to manage their stress. One in five Americans (20 percent) say they never engage in an activity to help relieve or manage their stress.

- The most commonly reported symptoms of stress in the past month include feeling nervous/anxious (35 percent), being irritable/angry (37 percent), feeling fatigued (32 percent), having a lack of interest/motivation (34 percent), being depressed/sad (32 percent), and feeling overwhelmed (32 percent).

- Many Americans say they engage in unhealthy behaviors because of stress, including eating too much/eating unhealthy foods (33 percent say they have done this in the past month because of stress).[2]

- Fewer than 5% of adults engage in the top health behaviors, and only 20% of adults are thriving.[3]

---

[1] American Psychological Association. 2017. "Stress in America: The State of Our Nation." November 1. Accessed June 30, 2019. www.stressinamerica.org.

[2] American Psychological Association. 2015. *Stress in America: Paying with our health.* February 4.Accessed June 30, 2019. https://www.apa.org/news/press/releases/stress/2014/stress-report.pdf.

[3] Berrigan, David, Kevin Dodd, Richard P Troiano, Susan M Krebs-Smith, and Rachel B Barbash. 2003. "Patterns of health behavior in U.S. adults." *Preventive Medicine* (Elsevier) 36 (5): 615-623.

Perhaps a more personal inventory would help.
Consider these descriptors ...

- ☐ Do you feel overwhelmed by the pace and load of work life?
- ☐ Are you considering cutting your work hours or changing jobs?
- ☐ Do you find it hard to fall asleep because of a racing mind?
- ☐ Do you check your phone immediately upon waking? Is it with you at the dinner table? Do you receive and respond to business emails or texts after work?
- ☐ Do you eat meals at your desk or in your car?
- ☐ Is your list of responsibilities for others so long that you never get to your own?
- ☐ Do you rely on coffee or other beverages or foods for quick energy?
- ☐ Do you depend on other drinks or food to decompress after a hard day?
- ☐ Do you feel uncomfortable with nothing to do?
- ☐ Have you given up hobbies?
- ☐ Do you give back vacation days?
- ☐ Do you have headaches or body aches that interrupt work?
- ☐ Do you have a chronic illness that has interrupted your perception of thriving?
- ☐ Are your personal and professional relationships suffering due to your choices or behaviors?

If you checked off even a couple of these, you are likely to benefit from this guide. I visited with a cardiologist attending my wellness workshop at a professional meeting. My description of the fast pace and intensity of life resonated with him. He is from Argentina. When he first came to the United States, he found it so strange that people would eat a meal in their car. The concept of "fast food" was not a part of his cultural experience in Argentina. But working and living in the US changes things. His head dropped as he confessed, "Now, I find myself eating in my car during my busiest days." So here we are … chasing the American dream … in some ways rewarded, challenged, and engaged, but also tired.

The indicators above are often evident in overachievers who are swept up in the pursuit of the American dream for prosperity and success that can be achieved by driving hard and fast. Not all of the above behaviors are bad. But it does help to reflect on how we are living and how our choices might contribute to our well-being. The idea of "hard work" is interesting and can be lived out in countless ways. Being a high achiever in itself is not a problem.

How you engage in "hard work" may be the difference between the sustainable success of an achiever and the steady decline in personal performance, personal health, and well-being of an overachiever. Shift Happens.

Resilience

> *"Persistence and resilience only come from having been given the chance to work through difficult problems."*
>
> –Gever Tulley

Resilience is a broad concept that includes the ability to withstand, adapt to, and recover from adversity and stress. It is multidimensional. We gain physical resilience when we work out at the gym. We test mental resilience in the pursuit of our education and job training. We reflect spiritual resilience when we align life choices and behaviors with our values and beliefs. The emotional domain, with emo̶t̶i̶o̶n̶a̶l̶ flexibility, positive outlook, and self-regulation, strongly impacts our ability to sustain our healthy living choices. Many feel untrained and ill-equipped with emotional skills or strategies to navigate the sometimes chaotic terrain of life.

DOMAINS OF RESILIENCE

Physical	Emotional	Spiritual	Mental
Physical flexibility	Emotional flexibility	Spiritual flexibility	Mental flexibility
Endurance	Positive Outlook	Commitment to values	Attention span
Strength	Self-regulation	Tolerance of others	Ability to focus

Resilience is a target for self-care that mobilizes the power to adapt and flourish. People endure unprecedented levels of stress in life and work that drain mental, physical, emotional, and spiritual resilience, making it difficult to pursue and achieve wellness. Our best intentions can get derailed if we're ill-equipped to cope with the inevitable intrusion of stress in our lives. In fact, you may end up discouraged by repeated failed experiences to act on or sustain healthy choices.

The Brief Resilience Scale provided below provides important information to guide the course of your wellness plan.[4]

---

[4] Smith, B.W., J. Dalen, K. Wiggins, E. Tooley, P Christopher, and J. Bernard. 2008. "The Brief Resilience Scale: Assessing the ability to bounce back." *International Journal of Behavioral Medicine* 15: 194-200.

Brief Resilience Scale

 Please complete this brief inventory for your current resilience experience and record your score below.

1. I tend to bounce back quickly after hard times.

Strongly Disagree = 1 Disagree = 2 Neutral = 3 Agree = 4 Strongly Agree = 5

2. I have a hard time making it through stressful events.

Strongly Disagree = 5 Disagree = 4 Neutral = 3 Agree = 2 Strongly Agree = 1

3. It does not take me long to recover from a stressful event.

Strongly Disagree = 1 Disagree = 2 Neutral = 3 Agree = 4 Strongly Agree = 5

4. It is hard for me to snap back when something bad happens.

Strongly Disagree = 5 Disagree = 4 Neutral = 3 Agree = 2 Strongly Agree = 1

5. I usually come through difficult times with little trouble.

Strongly Disagree = 1 Disagree = 2 Neutral = 3 Agree = 4 Strongly Agree = 5

6. I tend to take a long time to get over setbacks in my life.

Strongly Disagree = 5 Disagree = 4 Neutral = 3 Agree = 2 Strongly Agree = 1

Scoring: Add the value (1–5) of your responses for all six items, creating a range from 6–30. Divide the sum by the total number of questions answered (6) for your final score.

Total Score =

Divide Total Score by 6 =

BRS Score	Interpretation
1.00 - 2.99	Low Resilience
3.0 - 4.3	Medium Resilience
4.31 - 5.0	High Resilience

Even if you score high in resilience, that does not exclude you benefiting from this work. Many of my clients actually score medium to high in resilience, yet they perceive that they are somehow lacking because life feels so out of balance, overwhelming, or off-track.

Another approach to describing resilience relates to how it's being applied:

Bounce Back	Bounce back easily from setbacks.
Prepare	Having a self-care/self-regulation plan in place for difficult moments, situations, or relationships.
Sustain	Sustain good physical and emotional health when under constant pressure.
Cope	Cope with ongoing disruptive change.
Overcome	Overcome adversities.
Change	Change to a new way of working or living when an old way is no longer possible or sustainable.
Do	Do all this without acting in a dysfunctional or harmful manner.

The real challenge involves resisting **dysfunctional or harmful means of coping.** We may make choices or behave in ways that are not optimal for ourselves, our work, or relationships. I had one client who consulted their physician regarding symptoms that he worried were the result of significant anxiety or heart issues. As it turns out, his symptoms were related to excessive caffeine consumption that was helping him meet his strenuous workload.

Sometimes on my way home from a challenging day of work, I'm tempted to stop at a gas station to purchase some of their arsenal of energy support for people. My vice is sugar, and I'm tempted to reward my hard day with a sweet treat. Growing up, my dad often gifted me a candy bar after a sporting event or academic achievement.

I fondly remember the days of my youth when a stressful day was being denied outdoor recess because of the weather! I also remember returning home after elementary school, watching *Scooby-Doo* on TV with my mom in the kitchen making dinner, while I relaxed and enjoyed a treat gifted to me with love. I recognize that buying myself a treat simply connected me to the love, comfort, and relaxation I experienced when I was ten years old. Is a sugary treat really my only option to achieve those ends? No.

Life as an adult is definitely more complex. The stakes are higher, the days longer, and the responsibilities heavier. Not only are my days more rigorous, but now I'm the loving parent who wants to make a healthy meal and extend a gesture of love to my children. How do any of us extend love when our own inner reserve is empty?

I've since discovered a variety of healthy options to support my well-being through strenuous days. Most recognize the discomfort and feeling that you're "losing yourself" during a stressful stint of life. By engaging in your personal growth, you can begin to unravel your own motivations and start shifting towards healthier coping strategies that facilitate well-being. It took a lot of experimentation to override my strong urge to use sugar to support my mood and energy. Resilience strategies regulate energy and mood so you can confidently and effectively engage in stressful work environments and still bring your best self home to those you love the most.

Flow versus Flood

Mihaly Csikszentmihalyi, the author of *Flow*, studied states in which people report feelings of concentration and deep enjoyment.[5] His research revealed that what makes an experience genuinely satisfying is "flow"—a state of concentration so focused that it amounts to complete absorption in an activity and results in the achievement of an ideal state of happiness. *Flow* has become the classic work on happiness and was a major contribution to contemporary psychology. It describes a state that can truly elevate performance and satisfaction. It can feel good and be productive and efficient—until it's not.

At what point does the flow of being absorbed in your work grow into a flood with negative consequences? High achievers know and experience flow. And overachievers are vulnerable to losing the vitality of flow when they lose the reins on their passion, purpose, and drive.

The idea of "hard work" is interesting and can be lived out in countless ways. Being a high achiever in itself is not a problem. ***How*** you engage in "hard work" may be the difference between the sustainable success of an achiever and the steady decline in personal performance, health, and well-being that may impact the overachiever.

Overachievers often acclimate to a very accelerated pace in life and work. Absorption in work can grow from minutes into hours. Missed meetings, social commitments, or a meal (or two) are collateral damage to uninterrupted engagement. Others can sit or stand in awkward positions for crazy amounts of time, completely absorbed in their task or challenge. Some become so deeply engaged in a project on the computer that hours pass without registering. These behaviors may be appropriate at times. But they are becoming the norm.

---

[5]   Nakamura, Jeanne, and Mihaly Csikszentmihalyi. 2009. "Flow Theory and Research." In *The Oxford Handbook of Positive Psychology*, by Shane, J. Lopez and C.R. Snyder, 195-206. Oxford: Oxford University Press.

The "I'm on a roll" perception convinces people that a break from this flow state interrupts productivity, or they fear not having the energy or ability to get back on track. The decision to remain engaged without a break may be productive, but likely, at a cost. Mental capacity can fatigue (just like the body) and lead to mistakes or clouded thinking. Uninterrupted intense engagement can lead to significant orthopedic or other physical issues that eventually require medical attention.

My husband, a cardiologist, is often caught up in the flow state. By the nature of his long hours of education and training, he's enjoyed the absorption of engaging his interest, pursuing a challenge, applying his skills, and experiencing the sense of accomplishment that is the reward of hard work. I've also witnessed his experience of "flow" turning to "flood" as the momentum of drive and pursuit of achievement leave no space for self-awareness or self-care. His ability to flow through several hours of work on call led him to neglect sensations of hunger or fatigue. This state of "hangry," as we call it in our house, is a combination of hungry and angry. While he may have been productive when he was in the flow, it had the unintended consequences of disrupting relationships with family and often resulted in expedient but not always healthy food choices.

This ability to work without rest builds resilience for sure. Many professions train under stressful conditions to produce a resilient workforce. In flow, when individuals have the skills, interest, and sense of accomplishment to reward them, they can work incredibly long stints without rest. But without space for recuperation or rest, there comes a tipping point of diminishing returns. For some, they can become resilient to a fault.

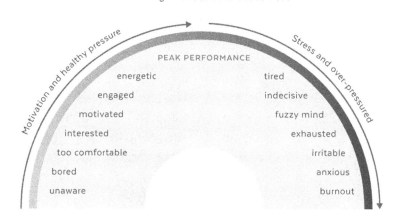

THE STRESS ARC
maintaining motivation without burnout

Stress occurs when perceived pressure on an individual
exceeds ability to maintain resilience.

Resilient to a Fault

Stress, burnout, compassion fatigue, and emotional exhaustion are rampant in today's work culture and afflict people from a variety of professional disciplines and stations of life. Work cultures are increasing the pace and intensity of the workday, and the human capital is paying the price. The workday itself is creeping into personal time. Fueled by incredible resilience, in an effort to maintain peak performance, many high achievers give up days off, work through weekends and vacations, and take work home. They skip meals, dentist or doctor appointments, or family events in service of their work. Technology is keeping people tethered to work in ways unimaginable a decade ago. And it's easy to experience an unhealthy separation from the natural world, loved ones, and even yourself. People are wearier than ever. And they're vulnerable.

Young adulthood is particularly challenging. Investment is made to build careers and families, and life gets more complex. Parents, in particular, report higher average stress levels than nonparents.[6] They work exhaustively to satisfy the many obligations that exist in their lives ... likely growing their resilience ... to a fault.

Consider this familiar scenario:

> James and Briana's day starts before the crack of dawn. He prepares lunches for kids and Briana. She preps their dinner. James has the longer commute ... traveling thirty-five minutes (on a good day) in heavy traffic. They both put in an overly full day of work. Briana uses her break to arrange doctor appointments for her aging parents. James crams a workout in over lunch to fend off his borderline hypertension. Together, they juggle the kids' after-school activities, needs of ailing parents, and household errands in the little time they have after work. Briana feels guilty having a gym membership. She hasn't been able to attend her cycle class for a month. Dinner is a whirlwind. Kids are bathed, read to, and put to bed. Though exhausted, there's mounting laundry, dishes, taxes, pet care, and prep for a work meeting the next day. Sleep comes easy for James. Briana lies in bed, exhausted, but unable to stop her racing mind ... dreading the restart of it all in less than 6 hours.

This scenario could easily be upset by an unexpected personal life crisis or an unsupportive work environment where increased effort is met with unrelenting task loading, understaffing, lack of appreciation, diminished resources, or unrecognized accomplishments. Such crises become tipping points that shift lives from just manageable to

---

[6]   American Psychological Association. 2015. *Stress in America: Paying with our health.* February 4.Accessed June 30, 2019.
https://www.apa.org/news/press/releases/stress/2014/stress-report.pdf.

overwhelming. The James and Brianas of the world are committed to making ends meet, engaging with kids, excelling at work, and caring for parents. They're exhausted and struggling, possibly because they've lost touch with the higher purpose that inspires what they do and why.

Stretching the workforce to sometimes unreasonable limits is prevalent across disciplines. Education, business, industry, and government can all fall prey to the insidious creep of stressing their human capital. Luckily, the conversation is shifting from one where wellness and resilience are considered employee perks to one where they are professional responsibilities to support the sustainability of the workforce in order to meet the mission of organizations.

Driven and dedicated lifestyles are a complex mix of necessity, devotion, expectation, and habit. Sadly, being overcommitted and stressed out is often considered a badge of honor or rite of passage in American work culture, and no one is immune from this pressure. The employed, the self-employed, volunteers, and homemakers are all vulnerable. Selflessness is often perceived as virtuous, while tending to personal needs is seen as weak or selfish.

Many take the resilience inventory at the start of this chapter and they score medium to high. So what gives? They think they need to be **more resilient.** What they quickly realize is that without pause for proper rest, physical nourishment, and emotional support or regulation, their resilience can become an Achilles' heel.

I've worked with two types of high achievers who are at particular risk for burnout. They have a tendency to overachieve or are resilient to a fault:

- "Expert" achievers
- "Have-it-all" achievers

Experts streamline their focus and direct energy and resources towards a specific goal, field, subject, or skill. The energy and passion of young adulthood fuel the development of this work ethic while the individual is still relatively free from the complexities of life, such as marriage, children, aging parents, or expanding financial pressures.

Careers advance, and compensation improves along this path. Awards are received, and great work is done. But choices lead to habits, and habits have consequences. Sometimes there is a price to pay for such a narrow pursuit of excellence. Individuals experience discontent, dis-ease, or damaged relationships.

"Have-it-all" achievers have their own unique approach. These folks don't "dabble" in a variety of areas, they tirelessly pursue excellence in everything they do with a "have-it-all" mentality. This style also develops early in life. Youth today are pressured into academic, extracurricular, and volunteer commitments that reinforce an overachiever mindset. This conditioning stretches into college and early career development years.

In addition to commitments toward career advancement, young and resilient bodies often enjoy volunteering, engaging in vigorous exercise, physical competition, and high-energy social activities. Think color runs, advocacy work, dance clubs, and the latest fitness craze. Just reminiscing about this phase of life raises my own energy level—what a joy this time of life can be! But again, behaviors become habits.

Caution: Behaviors can become habits. And habits are not easily changed. As the complexities of life pile on, commitments increase, the body ages, and like it or not, the ability to withstand stress changes.

Whether you're a young executive trying to leave your mark, a new nurse or medical resident trying to apply years of education to the sometimes insane pace of medicine, or a new parent juggling work and family commitments, the early years of life and career can be grueling.

Midlife offers its own version of complexity. And retirement isn't always a piece of cake either. Conditioned high achievers can really struggle when retirement affords them an abundance of free time.

> Elevating self-care to a personal and professional responsibility can reduce or alleviate much of the stress and strain that accompanies the various stages of life.

Let me emphasize again ... being a high achiever is not the problem. Whether driven toward too narrow a focus or spread too thin, the challenge comes not from being a high achiever but from making an incessantly ramped up pursuit of life and success a habit. By neglecting the restorative power of rest and self-care, individuals create habits that, over time, can deteriorate the body, mind, and spirit. Such unchecked habits can become toxic lifestyles down the road. And there is definitely little capacity for the unplanned events that often interrupt life.

Being passionate and driven in your work is a strength. Yet it's a fire that needs to be controlled. Putting all your energy into one dimension of your well-being impacts your life in complex ways. If work commands your time and energy, sleep may be interrupted, relationships may be strained, play is budged out, and meaning and purpose may become clouded.

Fast foods meet the need for a fast-paced life. Struggling to endure a busy day, overachievers may succumb to the temptation of a variety of energy-boosting products and behaviors to meet commitments. Energy may be fueled by coffee, smoking, or sugary foods and drinks that are easily found in break rooms or strategically placed at most store checkouts. It is no surprise that coffee shops and convenience stores with caffeine, sugar, and smokes are on every corner.

Once these high-octane products and activities rocket people through an overly packed day, downregulating becomes a new target. Sometimes alcohol, TV, electronic games, books, or other forms of escapism fill what little time is left in a draining day. It's no surprise, then, that the same adrenaline-seeking, cortisol-flooded, caffeine-, sugar-, or nicotine-fueled overachievers suffer from interrupted sleep! The one built-in restorative practice designed to replenish energy, heal the body, rest the mind, and restore mood is sacrificed in service to work.

Both the "Expert" and the "Have-it-all" overachievers may describe their pursuit as what they love. But even doing too much of what you love can turn a desirable flow state into a flood. The symptoms of flood moments in life can be very unsettling. A racing mind can keep you up at night. Headaches, gut issues, or a racing heart can raise concern for health. It's not uncommon for clients to seek physician guidance due to health complaints before being referred for stress management and self-regulation skill development.

People with autoimmune symptoms or disease, sleep disturbance issues, anger management, anxiety, and depression can all benefit from wellness strategies that support self-care and stress management. In addition to medical treatment, these conditions benefit from managing the stress that is epidemic in life today.

The "Expert" and "Have-it-All" achievers strive for—and often achieve—success through virtues like **dedication, discipline,** and **drive.** These same virtues can be applied to personal growth and resilience skill development. Thriving in life and work becomes achievable and sustainable when **dedication** to self-care is seen as a personal and professional responsibility. **Discipline** is used to practice necessary self-care skills, and **drive** is tempered with self-regulation that allows you to live another day to execute at peak performance.

The Mindful Pause process has helped countless individuals incorporate restorative elements into their lives. A bank executive developed better ways to manage stress; a doctor lost weight to regulate blood pressure; and several nurses, EMTs, and physician assistants addressed perfectionist habits that threatened important relationships. Additionally, government employees, cancer survivors, managers, domestic engineers, college students, young parents, and others have creatively integrated the Mindful Pause process into their lives in order to live their best life vision.

In fact, you may surprise yourself at the level of performance that you can enjoy by living an intentional life that prioritizes self-care in the pursuit of excellence.

Surviving Adversity

A disciplined life of self-care and a devoted self-regulation practice does not guard one from upset in life. Life always has the potential to throw a curveball that catches you off guard. Adversity, though not desirable, is effective at prompting personal growth. People can experience profound growth when living with a life-threatening illness. People in the aftermath of divorce, the loss of a child, or amid the stress of career transitions discover strengths not previously known. So even if you have enjoyed your own version of pursuit of excellence without burnout, life happens. Anyone can be caught in unfamiliar territory, thrown off balance, or knocked out of whack by unexpected life events.

This journey is for all those who extend themselves beyond reasonable limits and are vulnerable to an imbalance and fatigue that comes with either too narrow a life focus or one so fractured and overcommitted that they find themselves on a path of burnout and fatigue.

Those who find themselves at a fork in the road without a clear sense of what to do next can find clarity. When life pulls the rug out from underneath you, and you need a path to a new way of living and being, resilience gives you stability to cope with change. Not all the coping mechanisms previously mentioned are uniformly bad. But in the absence of a robust and holistic wellness plan that includes self-care and resilience skills, some coping strategies can accelerate the risk of burnout, anxiety, compassion fatigue, disrupted relationships at work and in families, or one of many stress-induced symptoms that plague people today.

 Reflect

- What are your thoughts regarding your Resilience score?
- In what ways do you recognize yourself in the "achiever" mindsets?
- What coping "habits" poorly impact your health?

Chapter 2

Your Inner Compass

Are You Ready?

There are many stages of readiness in the change process. Are you just thinking about change? Is someone else telling you that you should change? Or are you all in and ready to go but not sure where or how to start? Clarity around readiness helps set appropriate goals. This is where working with a coach can be very helpful. Coaches are trained to recognize readiness and match goals appropriately. This is important for effective behavior change.

Shortly after college, I took a job as the Director of Fitness at a YWCA. As part of that role, I had to complete my water safety instructor training. One of the testing requirements included treading water for five minutes carrying a five-pound brick. I had competed in college basketball, run a marathon, and was currently teaching several fitness classes a week. While not an exceptional swimmer, I was a competent swimmer and felt like this would be an easy pass. The instructor asked if I would like some tips before taking the test. I declined. My youth and ego bolstered my confidence but blocked any willingness to be open to support. So in the water I went. Treading and ready for the challenge, he handed me the brick. The brick was heavier than I expected. It was clear I needed to work hard to keep above water. My legs went faster

... and faster ... and my breathing picked up to match my exertion. For about five seconds, I kept this up. Then I was under. Done. Test over. Clinging to the pool wall, shocked and out of breath, my instructor kindly asked, "Would you like that advice now?"

Readiness is a curious thing. Often, by the time people seek help, they have sunk underwater enough times that they are more than ready. Life can get difficult. Some find that familiar or habituated coping strategies no longer bring relief. This could simply come about with age.

For example, some clients have used vigorous exercise for stress relief but reach a point in life where intense movement is no longer the proper remedy. Or a lifetime of ineffective or destructive choices finally catch up and are eroding health, relationships, or performance at work. At this tipping point or sinking point, as in my example, many are ready to seek change.

Curious about what happened next with the brick test? The instructor just smiled with amusement, knowing that my failure was a great teachable moment. He explained the nugget of wisdom in working smarter, not harder. My racing legs and quick, shallow breathing only made my body heavier and fatigued the resources of my breath and leg strength too quickly. He pointed out that relaxing and laying back slightly to disperse my body weight across the surface would allow my lungs to inflate and act as a buoy to suspend not only my body but the five-pound brick as well. Equipped with this simple strategy, the seemingly impossible five-minute target became a target easily within my reach. Stop racing, breathe deeply, think strategically, and choose success.

Permission for Self-Care

Self-care is never a selfish act.

–Parker Palmer

Self-care is the practice of taking an active role in protecting one's well-being and happiness, particularly during periods of stress. Holistic self-care includes attention to the physical, mental, spiritual, and emotional domains.

> "I need to make me a priority, but it's not easy. It takes commitment and effort. I'm good at helping others, but make excuses when it comes to me (she sighs). Or maybe I'm simply just too tired."
>
> –Kim, departmental director in urban hospital, wife, and mother.

Kim describes a common scenario. Prioritizing self-care may be new, unfamiliar, or undervalued. First and foremost, it is important to recognize that a self-care mindset is NOT selfish, self-indulgent, pampering, or a luxury. Self-care IS a personal and professional responsibility. It's a necessary skill for anyone who wants to maintain a satisfying and sustainable engagement in life, work, and relationships.

Developing holistic self-care habits is as relevant and essential as any other skill set that you train for in life and work. As such, it cannot wait until that day off, weekend, or vacation that you never take. It is important to incorporate self-care habits throughout each day.

Whether you teach, heal, sell, counsel, manage, or parent, you are likely to have invested time, money, and training into activities that help you excel at your work. Unfortunately, few of the busy and overcommitted give themselves permission to include self-care in their financial or time budget.

Jane, who commutes an hour (one-way) to work as a busy nurse executive, had this to say about self-care:

> "I want to do self-care without guilt and not worry about what other people might think. I strongly value doing a really good job. I'm driven. Other's opinions are very important to me. I want to find balance with this commitment and my own commitment to my self-care. I want to learn to manage my perfectionist tendencies and acquire the skills to override habits with new choices."
>
> She goes on to describe, "It was difficult for me to reach out for help, but after I did, I am glad I did. I have found this experience a good one. It is a great opportunity to learn more about myself and to learn how to truly change so I can believe in the statement that self-care is not a selfish act."

Jane is also a parent of adult children. So she quickly recognized that her commitment to self-care was not a selfish act but a commitment to preserving her health and well-being so that she can enjoy and be present for her growing family. In her story, there are two important indicators:

- First, she has a history of prioritizing her work and commitments to others ahead of herself. This is a habit that will take practice to change.

- Second, you can hear her values. She values hard work. But she also values her health and her family relationships. She shared excitement for upcoming weddings for her daughters and her wish to be healthy and vibrant to enjoy the next phase of life.

By identifying her motivations, the power of permission grew stronger, and the distraction of others' expectations and unreasonable boundaries started to fade. Shift Happens.

Jane and Kim are not alone. Many struggle with reframing their perception of self-care. When we take a look at how and where we invest our time, energy, and resources (including money), self-care is often low on the list. Time is dedicated to work, children, extended family, community, and more. Energy is spent from start to finish "doing" for others, which leaves little time for the "beingness" that restores and heals the doer. And it's not uncommon to prioritize financial resources for maintenance on our cars, lawns, and home but neglect the maintenance of our own personal health.

Rest and recovery are important elements of self-care. There is a widespread loss of appreciation for rest as part of the natural cycle of life, and choices for coping are often life-draining instead of life-giving. I met a woman who owned a small jewelry shop where she sold her craft. We chatted while I browsed through her treasures.

Her life was much different now as an artist. She had grown up on a farm where work started at dawn and didn't end until dusk. If you rested, you were lazy and unproductive. In her case, besides stopping to eat a meal, smoking was the only culturally permissible break. Smoking isn't the only coping behavior that threatens health and well-being. A variety of foods or entertainment may provide comfort or energy but threaten vitality or long-term health. As an essential professional skill, we must create environments and systems that support rest and recovery.

An abundance of appropriate self-care choices exist that enhance life, mood, and energy. Walking in nature, art, gardening, or reading are common choices. But people find incredibly unique choices for self-care. I heard a story on public radio of a police chief who rose at the crack of dawn to watch bees leave their hive for work.

The options are countless. But your busy life has to *stop* in order to hear, feel, and know how you are uniquely being called to restore yourself. A doctor who has been on her feet all day may need to sit with her feet up and read a book. For an accountant who's been stuck at her desk all day, rest may be a restorative walk outside.

If you take nothing else away from this book, it is my hope that you gain a greater appreciation for building in "stops" for self-care that restore your body, clear your mind, and strengthen your spirit. And in doing so, you restore yourself so that you bring your best self into all the meaningful ways you engage in life. How often do you need to practice self-care? How often do you eat? Wellness is a lifestyle. Self-care is essential. And you are worth your best effort. Permission granted.

I want to take a moment to guide you through a visualization of what holistic well-being might look and feel like if you give yourself permission.

 Imagine yourself waking before your alarm—well-rested with a sense of eagerness to start your day. Your morning ritual gives you time to wake up and align your intentions in body, mind, and spirit. See yourself living into a day of engaging work, nourishing food and drink, healthy relationships, movement, and joy. You feel grounded in healthy habits, a growing sense of purpose and satisfaction with work and relationships, and gifted with a strong sense of self-control. You meet frustrations with stability and ease and recover quickly from disappointment. With regular breaks, you have plenty of energy to be productive at work and still have time and energy to engage with family, friends, or your community in ways that enrich your life. You take time for a nourishing meal and, at the close of your day, engage in an evening ritual that relaxes your body and quiets your mind. Your sleep comes easy.

Sound nice? Achievable? How big is the gap between where you are now and where you want to be? Any gap you feel can be exacerbated by the pace and intensity of life. A fast-paced, driven life slowly erodes satisfaction and dulls your vision of a vital life. Use the Mindful

Pause to *Stop, Breathe,* give space to *Think* about your unique needs and values, and then *Choose* to give yourself permission to prioritize self-care.

CLIENT CASE STUDY: PERMISSION FOR SELF-CARE

Situation

Kim, accreditation and regulatory compliance program manager in a large urban hospital setting, was feeling overwhelmed at work and tired all the time despite getting enough sleep.

Desired Outcome

- Improve self-regulation of mood and energy

Kim's Impactful Program Elements

- Movement
- Meditation
- Mindful Pause

Kim's Results

When asked at a weekly check-in what she was most proud of, Kim said, "I took the time for me. Kids and husband were gone. Spent some time with myself and felt amazing!" Kim gave herself permission to schedule time each day for movement and meditation.

She embraced the invitation to try new activities. She started getting up at 5 am and walking before work. She practiced Mindful Pause each morning and evening and sometimes throughout the day. Her commitments were "a priority and a necessity."

"I'm realizing I need a lot of practice. Takes me a really long time to get 'in the zone'—much more difficult than I anticipated. This past week has been a lot of self- reflection. Our last session was very eye-opening for me. I need the practice, as this does not come easy or naturally for me. I have a long way to go, but that's okay. I just feel really blessed that I am finally learning the tools that can help me. Now is the time! I am succeeding because I am changing my mindset and seeing the importance of taking time for me and self-reflection. I'm feeling less stuck and more in control of my life."

Kim's story gives us an honest understanding of how something can be simple but not easy. The practices that she was integrating were not overly time-consuming or challenging. The real work came in overriding old habits.

Stories illustrate strengths, beliefs, and values. I experienced a strong affirmation about the importance of self-care after facilitating a wellness retreat.

On a beautiful fall Sunday afternoon, I hosted a wellness retreat at our state park. It was peak season, and the landscape was adorned with a tapestry of fall colors. A group of about 25 had gathered in the lodge for an afternoon to practice self-care and resilience-building skills. We explored meditation, mindfulness, gentle yoga, a nature walk, and crafted wellness visions all in a beautiful setting unplugged from technology.

I used the monarch butterfly as inspiration for this retreat. The story of the monarch butterfly begins on a particular tree that grows on a particular mountain range in Mexico that serves as the birthplace for this remarkable species. Four generations of monarch travel north through the summer months. The late summer monarch, or "super monarch," as it is called, faces the amazing challenge of flying the thousands of miles back to its home. So how do the super monarchs know where to go? They have never been to Mexico. Their parents or grandparents have never been to Mexico. How is this possible?

> *Inside each of us, there is a marvelous compass which greatly favors life, freedom and vitality.*
>
> –Bryant McGill

Science cannot yet fully explain this mystery. It is thought that their "inner compass" somehow draws them to the destination of their calling.

We do know that the monarch's existence is in jeopardy. Numbers have been falling dramatically in recent decades. The monarch butterfly is close to being placed on the endangered or threatened species list. Many suspect that toxins in the environment, including air and possibly noise pollution, may contribute. Others surmise that landscape and roadside maintenance choices like mowing and using herbicides threaten their food supply.

The monarch is not the only species threatened by our increasingly toxic environments. An alarming number of Americans face unprecedented levels of stress in their personal and professional lives. These unhealthy environments can interrupt our wellness and ability to thrive. Threats include toxins in our food supply, the environment, relationships, and even the thoughts we think.

I used the monarch to encourage attendees to explore the importance of going on a retreat to tap into their own "inner compass" and then create a wellness vision that takes them to their own "Mexico"—the place where they can regenerate their own life story.

At the conclusion of the retreat, participants had their own wellness vision (their Mexico) and an origami butterfly to remind them of their commitment.

On the morning following the retreat, I woke early and went for a run. It was another beautiful fall day. As I approached my house at the end of my run, a monarch came and landed on my arm! No lie! She stayed with me for about 10 minutes. I left the driveway and walked to my side garden and sat down with her still resting on my forearm. She seemed to be gently stretching her wings by lightly floating them up and down. She was also probing my skin. I suspect that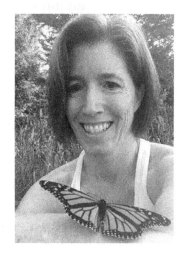

she was enjoying the salt that was the result of the sweat from my run. So we sat there and shared a moment. Want to know what she taught me? Her presence affirmed two things:

Lesson #1: Self-Care is Essential

She was obviously one of the super monarchs embarking on the journey of a lifetime. But she took time to rest, nourish herself, and stretch. I hope that you, like my butterfly friend, can take a moment to rest and nourish yourself with the wisdom and strategies that help so many discover their Mexico.

Lesson #2: Life is a Miracle

There are two kinds of people in the world. Those who don't believe in miracles. And those who believe everything is a miracle.

–Popular Wisdom

Everything is a miracle. *You* are a miracle. Your wellness journey towards your meaningful and rewarding life will amaze you with its own miracles. It's not uncommon for people to experience amazing synchronicities when they engage in intentional living. They're shocked when shortly after naming a desire for love, that love shows up in unpredictable ways. Or, when gently redirecting attention toward the existence of goodness and blessing in life, their anxiety, grief, or physical discomforts wondrously lessen.

Follow the cairns and journey on.

To see a video I captured of my monarch friend, visit the resources page of my website: GuidedResilience.com

Chapter 3
Your Holistic Well-Being

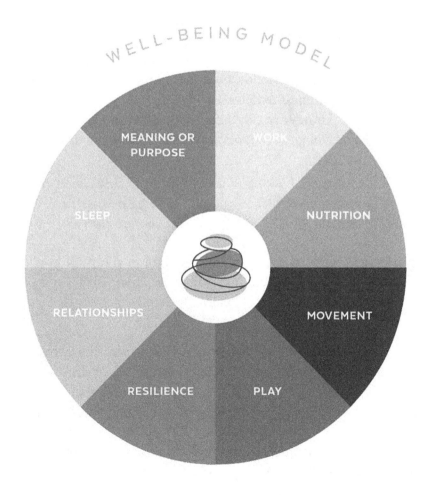

WELL-BEING MODEL

MEANING OR PURPOSE

WORK

SLEEP

NUTRITION

RELATIONSHIPS

MOVEMENT

RESILIENCE

PLAY

The word **holistic** comes from the Greek word *holos,* meaning "entire" or "all." It contains the dimensions that are relevant and important for clients seeking life satisfaction throughout varying seasons of life. Each dimension contributes to a holistic vision of your life and is inextricably linked to the other dimensions.

Maintaining a holistic lens is essential to well-being. It's easy when life gets challenging or busy to become myopic in our life focus. For example, being consumed with an intense work project or parenting young children may make your work dimension very full and mostly satisfying, but perhaps it depletes your sleep.

While directing energy to one dimension may be necessary for periods of time, holism dictates that everything is interrelated, and choices have costs. As a result, a deficit in sleep can negatively impact other areas and decrease satisfaction overall. Taking a pause can give you the space and awareness to determine what sources provide vitality or depletion. This knowledge can then give insight into how you should approach change in areas that matter most to you at the time.

 So let's STOP and consider your holistic well-being. You can download a worksheet and instructions from my website: GuidedResilience.com

I encourage you to get out your crayons or markers. If you don't have any, this may be an action step in your future! Play is one of the dimensions of well-being, and coloring is a simple activity that lets you feel playful and creative.

One point to consider as you complete your assessment: the "Movement" dimension invites you to take a broad perspective of the movement you get throughout a day (not just exercise from a workout). Physical movement is essential to health. Some people regularly get 30 minutes of moderate to vigorous exercise most days of the week but spend an additional 10 hours of the day sitting in front of a computer for work. Inactivity erodes vitality. Assess yourself honestly.

Once completed, take a look at your circle. What do you see? Record a couple of thoughts in your journal or on your worksheet.

Now, look at what you wrote. Did your reflection focus on the areas that are depleted? Most people notice deficits. "This is a really sad wheel." Or, "I have a lot to work on." This reaction is not wrong. It just illustrates the strong inclination for a negativity bias. Negativity bias is a natural human tendency and one that is often trained and reinforced in our work. We look for what's wrong ... and try to fix it.

Teachers correct papers. Mechanics fix machines. Managers improve inefficiencies. Doctors and nurses diagnose illness and injury and work to heal it. This only becomes problematic if we lose the ability, and it's easy to do, to recognize and savor all that is good. Leaving a day of work with a negativity lens leads you to miss the beautiful sky and only notice the potholes on your path. Or instead of seeing people on sidewalks as interesting, you see them more as problems to solve.

Keep this exercise handy. It is often one of the most impactful exercises that my clients reflect upon and can be revisited during the varying seasons of life.

The Illustrious "Work/Life Balance"

We hear a lot about work/life balance. What does it mean to bring "balance" to your wheel? Balance suggests equilibrium. Equilibrium may not equate to satisfaction. Remember the reference to "flow versus flood"? I have met many clients who succumb to a flood in an effort to bring equilibrium to their wheel. They exhaust themselves in an effort to satisfy all the "shoulds." I *should* be exercising more. I *should* be eating better.

I frequently remind my clients that for lasting change, we need to stop *"shoulding"* on ourselves.

The well-being assessment is often eye-opening for clients. Clarity and intention grow out of self-reflection. This self-awareness exercise leads to conversations about priorities, gaps, desires, commitments, expectations, and hopes. Sometimes, clients are relieved to recognize the benefit when an area or two is depleted as a result of focusing on another dimension.

For example, an emergency department manager felt completely overwhelmed during the period for annual reviews. She had more than 70 employees that reported to her who were expecting thoughtful engagements to discuss their growing careers. It quickly became evident that certain domains of her well-being would be sacrificed for a time in service to this work.

She knew she would have to pass on some social engagements and likely lose a little sleep. But she was quickly able to defend this choice. A pause allowed her to recognize this choice was okay, given it would only be for a short push. Prioritizing work in this way brought deep satisfaction to her work domain as well as strengthening her sense of meaning/purpose. Considering her life holistically drew attention to the need to give herself permission for self-care through and after the push. She was able to look ahead in her calendar and make that self-care commitment.

Clarity and autonomous choice are key and can make all the difference in how you feel about your commitments.

A perfectly full and balanced wellness wheel is not necessarily the aim. What is important is *what matters to you.* While people easily identify the areas of their wheel that are diminished, explore the areas that are thriving and the perceived impact of the wheel as a whole in the experience of your life. It's important for you to discover where you are and engage in discerning and integrating self-care and resilience strategies for each particular season of life.

Where Am I Going? Creating Your MAP (My Action Plan)

Go confidently in the direction of your dreams! Live the life you've imagined.

–Henry David Thoreau

My Wellness Vision

Taking the time to create a clear wellness vision interrupts the tendency to just float through life and opens the door to the deeply satisfying experience of intentional living. More than balance, intentionality is what inspires vitality. What does your version of wellness look like? What are you doing in life? Who are you engaging with? What do you look like? How does this make you feel? Keep it real, but don't let perceived boundaries limit your thinking. Don't be afraid to think big—think wishes. This is a powerful exercise that often moves people beyond the "I should" of their plan into the "I want."

Take a moment now to put yourself in a comfortable place. Silence your phone. Take a couple of relaxation breaths. Envision your life five years from now with a sense of deep satisfaction in every dimension of your life. Try to see yourself living, moving, relating, and being in ways that are energizing and fulfilling. Savor that vision for a few moments.

41

Is your pen or pencil ready? Get out your journal or go to GuidedResilience.com to download your MAP worksheet on my resources page, then record your thoughts using the following tips for mapping your wellness vision.

Visions are best written in the present tense, making statements as if they are already your reality. A complete vision statement touches upon several of the dimensions from the well-being model. Sentences begin, "I am…" not "I will…." "I will" puts too big of a gap between you and your intention where you are vulnerable to falling into old habits.

Examples:

"At 50, I am enjoying ways to move and eat that support my energy and mood. My work is growing in new and exciting ways that keep me energized and engaged. I make time to enjoy my adult children and their growing families and enjoy an active lifestyle with my husband and friends. I intentionally stop, breathe, think, and choose to navigate confidently through personal challenges."

Or: "I am balancing a full life of work and parenting with intention and ease. I find creative ways to move and play that satisfy my needs and enrich my relationships with friends and family. I have healthy eating habits. I'm practicing a sleep hygiene routine that quiets my mind and restores my body so that my sleep comes easy."

Vision statements are free game. They are a place for you to express your intention creatively. One of my clients in recovery from cancer creatively expressed her vision for wanting to **THRIVE**, not just survive, with an acronym and bulleted list:

T aming the inner voice of doubt and fear about the future.

H ealthy eating with clean foods to support my body's ability to heal.

R esilient in the face of fear and doubt.

I nterested in new hobbies and friendships.

V alidating my new normal with compassion, optimism, and hope.

E nergy to engage in my life with passion and peace.

Others enjoy creative options like vision boarding, music, poetry, or art. Consider this your personal ad campaign. Companies spend billions of dollars putting images and catchy slogans in front of you to direct your behavior. Know why? Because it works! Your vision is meant to inspire you to action. Give yourself space and time to craft yours in a way that energizes and uplifts you.

Without a vision, you are likely to settle with where your current habits take you. Some seasons of life might need the familiarity of old habits. You will know the difference if you stop, breathe, think, and choose to consider what's in your head and in your heart. Holistic discernment is as much about feeling as it is thinking.

My Personal Strengths/Values

Personal strengths and values are sometimes difficult for clients to articulate. We are not accustomed to naming our strengths, yet it is one of the strongest contributors to successful and sustainable change. Knowing strengths is so important to a successful wellness plan, that I invite my clients to complete the VIA Survey of Character Strengths as part of their intake process. It is a simple self-assessment that takes less than 15 minutes, and the results show a rank order of your core values.

Most personality tests focus on negative and neutral traits, but the VIA Survey focuses on your best qualities. It was created under the direction of Dr. Martin Seligman, the "father of Positive Psychology" and author of *Flourish*.[7] It is regarded as a central tool of positive psychology and has been used in hundreds of research studies. It has been taken by over five million people in more than 190 countries.

If you decide to take the inventory, simply search for the VIA Survey of Character Strengths on the internet. Record your top five strengths for ongoing reference and integration into your plan.

In addition to the inventory, you can consider the following:

- What gives you pride?
- What qualities do you most appreciate about yourself?
- What do you value most about your life?
- What strengths can you draw on to help close the gap from where you are now to live into your vision?

3-Month Goals

With your vision in mind, you can begin to design intermediate goals to bring your vision closer to reality. To begin, I encourage clients to set 3-month goals. This time frame is long enough to make meaningful and informative progress toward establishing healthy habits yet is short enough to provoke a sense of urgency.

This is where you narrow your focus a bit and start to articulate SMART goals that move you in the direction of a desired outcome. SMART goals are: **Specific. Measurable. Action-based. Realistic. Time-based.**

---

[7] Seligman, Martin E. P. 2011. *Flourish*. New York: Free Press.

Here are some examples:

> **Desired Outcome:** Improve sleep.
>
> **SMART Goal:** I will unplug from electronics by 9 p.m. and journal about three blessings from my day before lights out at 10 p.m.

> **Desired Outcome:** To be fit and healthy.
>
> **SMART Goal:** At least three days every week, I will run three miles outdoors before work to enjoy nature.

Take time to brainstorm possibilities. Often, I find myself reining in my client's goals. It's very important to feel successful, especially early in the change process. Success builds success, so establishing thoughtful steps is crucial.

My Motivators

Too often, people are driven to change by the "should." "My boss thinks I need to learn to control my temper." Or, "My doctor says I need to lose weight and quit smoking." We all know what we **should** be doing. We don't need more evidence that exercise is good or that unrelenting stress is bad.

Much of the work in behavior change is bridging the gap between *knowing* and *doing*. If knowing was all it took, no doctor would be overweight, no nurse would smoke, and no counselor would be overwhelmed and stressed out. They know what they should be doing to be healthy, but **knowing and doing are two different things.**

Knowing is limited if it relies only on the capacity of our thinking mind. Knowing becomes powerful when connected to how we *feel*. When masterful at knowing and choosing an emotional landscape that aligns with values, doing becomes an affirmation of your best self.

This is **your** life, and you need to design it with your preferences, needs, and resources in mind. What are the benefits of making a change now? What is the driving force behind your desire to change? What do you treasure most about potential change?

These considerations keep you connected to the energy that will sustain your commitments. The clients who are the most successful implementing and sustaining change are the ones that unlock the secret to their true motivations.

How do you get to these true motivations? By feeling ... not just thinking. Your motivations emerge as you progress mindfully with an openness to experiment and learn.

My Challenges

Clients rarely need help with this section. This is just another example of how we often lead with our negativity bias. Challenges are often top of mind and are sometimes the impetus for engaging in change. Challenges can motivate or interrupt progress. Most readily identifiable challenges are external barriers like time, money, or equipment. But challenges may also be internal barriers like your own self-defeating thoughts, fears, doubts, or anxiety. Awareness of both can guide your action steps and experiments with change. Take a moment to record your thoughts around perceived challenges.

My Strategies

Consider the strategies and structures (people, resources, systems, and environments) needed to steer around or through challenges. What strategies may be effective in helping you realize your vision and meet your challenges? Feel free to brainstorm a bit here. Create a list that you can bring into the laboratory of your life experience.

This completes the My Action Plan (MAP).

 Review your plan. Read it out loud, if possible ... slowly ... to let each intention begin to take root in your body and mind. This is your MAP for a life that is deeply satisfying in meaning and purpose. Keep it close. Review it daily.

Consider where you will keep this plan. You might want to place a couple of copies strategically around, so it is easily accessible for motivation and clarity. Perhaps by your bedside or where you enjoy your morning coffee so you can recommit to your plan on a daily basis. Remember the old saying, "Out of sight, out of mind?" Help yourself out with as many reminders and cues as possible to keep you connected to your vision.

Chapter 4

SHIFT HAPPENS

Time and Stress

So what interrupts your commitment to a holistically satisfying life? Usually, time and stress are noted as challenges on most everyone's MAP. Let's explore a shift in our perspectives.

Time

A common barrier to prioritizing self-care is the belief that it has to take a lot of time. Finding the time may be challenging, but it's not impossible. This notion challenges us to consider priorities. Priorities can shift throughout life.

Self-reflection on priorities and values and an honest assessment of how you are spending time can help determine where and how you might carve out time to live into your MAP. Priorities can change, making it essential to practice a mindful approach to living that helps you adapt as needed.

Crucible or transitional moments in life have a way of shifting priorities. These moments may be uplifting times like getting married or starting a new job. Suddenly, we lose interest in binge-watching our favorite

TV show in order to spend time with a loved one or get a good night's sleep to show up refreshed at work. **When the "I want" overrides the "I should," we find the time.**

There can also be power in the "I have to." Priorities can sometimes be imposed by the threat of illness or moments of deep personal challenge like a divorce or the loss of a loved one or job. In a personal crisis, we may be forced to acknowledge the reality that holistic self-care is necessary.

I have worked with several cancer survivors who would never say cancer is desirable. But they do acknowledge that their journey shifted their priorities in a way that they would never want to give up. They felt motivated to make room in their life for enriching their relationships and life purpose, eating healthily, and moving and resting more.

For lasting change, however, the motivation of the "have to" eventually needs to transform into "want to." One cancer survivor I worked with struggled with feeling forced to give up her past food preferences in favor of whole foods. She found herself burdened by self-defeating thoughts of "why me?"

Her life was overhauled by her health crisis. She was investing her time, energy, and significant financial resources into supporting her health. One day, as she was shopping in a co-op for the organic and whole foods that were once absent from her diet, she noticed something. She was surrounded by young people—presumably healthy and active young people. And while she couldn't know their personal stories, she suspected that many of them were likely there by choice … not forced, as she had been feeling. This was the nudge she needed to shift her "have to" into "I want to" and made all the difference in habituating her new behaviors. With this shift, she no longer questioned the time or money she devoted to healthy behaviors.

Certainly, time management is a moving target in various seasons of life. Commitments evolve through early career, starting a family, career advancement, aging parents, and retirement. You set yourself up for success by bringing clarity to where and how you spend your time and energy and why.

It's not uncommon to fall into routines that simply haven't been challenged. When asked how she made progress with her self-care, a busy hospitalist and mother of two responded:

"Because I realize that daily self-care comes from ME ... the only sure way of getting consistent self-care is to make time for it every day."

My husband, Steve, is a collateral witness and sometimes target of my wellness coaching. His commitment to a career in medicine started back in college. He was a double major with a 4.0 in biology and chemistry. He once shared with me that he cut the strings on his guitar during finals so that he wouldn't be distracted from studies to play!

We started dating during our junior year of college. He insisted on two hours—at least—of studying before we could go out on a date. I was committed to including play, outdoor activity, healthy food, and sleep as part of my self-care routine. My grades were average when we met. We made a great pair. We were fortunate that as our relationship grew, we both positively influenced each other's use of time.

He found that the inclusion of some self-care added a greater sense of contentment to his rigorous pursuits. He learned he could play even a few minutes of guitar AND get great grades. He began practicing meditation and attending church with me to relieve the strenuous pursuit of a challenging professional career. Meanwhile, I benefitted from discovering that it wasn't so difficult to get great grades when I actually studied and still had time to play!

Self-reflection is essential in order to connect the dots, find meaning, and discover your "want to's." Even though it may take some time, it is not as much as you might expect, and the return on investment is definitely worth the effort.

Consider how you are spending your time. Identify some of your choices and reflect on how they align with your MAP. Give them a score, 1 being very low alignment with your vision and 10 being very strong alignment with your vision.

Stress

The term "stress" originated back in 1936 when Hans Seyle described it as the nonspecific response of the body to any demand for change. The physical response includes an increase in heart rate, blood pressure, muscle tension, breathing rate, and metabolism. Being nonspecific means stress can be experienced physically, mentally, and emotionally, and the same stressor can affect people differently.

Consider a group of friends on the downhill portion of a roller coaster ride. Of the four, three of them have huge smiles on their faces. One, in particular, is fearlessly enjoying the ride with hands thrown in the air, demonstrating a posture of trust in letting go. Contrast that with the fourth friend who is clutching the guard rail, eyes closed, and a pressured grimace on his face that suggests he'd like to compress time and end the ride more quickly.

The fearless friend is the kind of person who not only enjoyed the thrill of the ride, but she's likely to seek it out again … and again … perhaps repeat the ride ten times before calling it quits. Her friend, on the other hand, barely escaped losing his lunch on the ride and couldn't wait for it to be over. He's unlikely to return for a repeat experience—ever. In fact, even passing by the amusement park in the future gives him a post-traumatic stress response.

This scene effectively illustrates the difference between eustress and distress. Most people have to be reminded of the meaning of eustress. Eustress is generally considered beneficial stress, like moments on a roller coaster, giving a speech, competing in an event, or taking on a challenge. Generally considered positive, these are examples of how experiences that cause stress can also facilitate adaptation and growth. Stress definitely has a positive role to play in pursuing potential.

It isn't difficult to recognize the distress that accompanies threatening events. In fact, these are the events that often remain vivid in our memory. For example, most people can recall the awful sensations in the aftermath of barely escaping a traffic accident. Fear is likely the driver for fueling that very appropriate stress response. After the incident, your arms and legs quiver as a result of the stress hormones that flooded your body to assist emergently, perhaps even saving your life with its rapid response. Subsequently, it is likely that when you pass by that intersection in the future, you sense an apprehension or vigilance that warns you of potential danger. We remember distress.

Interestingly, the body responds in the same manner, whether experiencing eustress or distress. It's only our perception of the event that discriminates between the two. We might label eustress as "exciting," "challenging," or "awesome," like the roller coaster ride. Distress is more likely to be called "horrible," "traumatic," or "grueling," like avoiding a near accident—or a roller coaster ride! Changes in heart rate, breathing, blood pressure, muscle tension, and metabolism accompany most emotional experiences and often serve a necessary purpose.

But uninterrupted **chronic** stress—eustress or distress—is where people begin to suffer and deteriorate.

The most commonly reported sources of chronic stress include money (64 percent report that this is a very or somewhat significant source of stress), work (60 percent), the economy (49 percent), family responsibilities (47 percent), and personal health concerns (46 percent). [8]

---

[8] American Psychological Association. 2015. *Stress in America: Paying with our health.* February 4.Accessed June 30, 2019. https://www.apa.org/news/press/releases/stress/2014/stress-report.pdf.

Stress is unavoidable. Our perception of stress and what we reinforce can make a difference in the impact of stress on our life. With proper integration, stress can contribute to our personal growth and resilience. Considering the "Equally True" helps us make shifts happen.

Equally True

The possibility of witnessing the "equally true" is often overlooked and underappreciated. Research indicates that stress focuses attention, heightens senses, increases motivation, mobilizes energy, dampens fear, increases courage, enhances social connections, and helps your brain learn and grow.[9]

In a world too often dominated by judging outcomes as only success or failure, one can miss the rich opportunity to discover the equally true ... the sometimes unrecognized or underappreciated growth that comes out of difficult life events.

In a casual conversation with a colleague, we discussed her current life circumstances that were challenging in many ways. Her husband was recovering from cancer treatment, and they had recently moved his aging mother into their home. Her account of this time in her life was filled with gratitude, examples of friendship and support, and a deepening of her relationship with her husband. She noted that they both had grown individually and closer as a couple during this time.

Exploring the complete reality and impact of stress is essential. In addition to causing sometimes significant disruption in life, reflecting on stressful life circumstances can lead to resilience and growth by discovering the equally true. Shift Happens.

Leslie had a whirlwind weekend. She traveled three hours to set her daughter up at college (mostly eustress). While there, her mother

---

[9]   McGonigal, Kelly. 2015. *The Upside of Stress: why stress is good for you, and how to get good at it.* New York: Penguin Random House.

called and told her that her aged father had fallen and was hospitalized (distress). She then traveled for several hours to help her mother prepare for her father's return home.

This double whammy of stress left her feeling fatigued, far from resilient, and a bit guilty for taking time off of work to prioritize her parent's needs. But as we spoke, she began to recognize the equally true elements of the experience. It had increased her motivation, mobilized her energy, and enhanced her social connections. This lens helped her reframe the experience as a growth experience. The equally true elements also diminished the guilt she felt about missing work. It felt good to practice self-care by honoring her devotion to her family.

 Take a moment to recall a time that you experienced eustress and another time when you endured distress in some form. Reflect on and describe each experience and any rewards you gained. Be sure to include a pause to consider what might be equally true as a reward from the distressful experience.

Moments like these are worth recalling and then considering from the equally true perspective. Sometimes within these events, you'll discover clues about how you perform best. When you reflect on the equally true elements within these events, you also relive the experience from a positive lens that gives your body and mind the opportunity to rehearse the situations that lead to growth and energize your initiative to engage in the next challenge.

Your body, mind, and emotions communicate with you to help you understand your relationship to stressful life events.

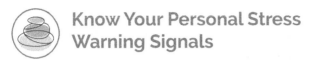

Know Your Personal Stress Warning Signals

What is your response to stress? Personal stress warning signals can show up in every dimension of well-being, including physical, mental, emotional, behavioral, spiritual, and relational. I like to view these signals as communication. Communication from these various dimensions is your ally, teacher, and friend as you navigate through life. This communication can come in the form of a whisper, yell, or two-by-four.

The whisper includes those earliest and most subtle signals that you're beginning to feel threatened or uncomfortable. Body "whispers" may be clenching of teeth or clamming up. It doesn't even have to be a stressful event. Check in while completing menial tasks like doing the dishes. Your body likely has a way of complaining that it would rather be out on an evening walk instead of stuck in a kitchen doing dishes.

If you ignore early signals of upset, your body may need to yell at you to get your attention. Fortunately, dishes really only take a few minutes and don't usually run the risk of causing prolonged stress. But other times, you may easily move through advancing stress warning signals.

When I'm working on a presentation on my computer, I can get lost in thought. I may clench my teeth as I press through the work. I actually enjoy this work, but the intensity of my focus carries into my body. If I don't take a break, my teeth clenching can turn into neck and shoulder tension and pain from my extended time at the computer. My body finds a way to yell at me.

Sometimes, people (myself included) are well trained to ignore the yell. Perhaps a deadline or just the flow of the work postpones good self-care. But your body has clever ways to get what it needs. And if it is experiencing too much neglect, life can come through with the two-by-four. A two-by-four moment may be an illness, injury, or breakdown.

Repeated work at my computer without proper stretching or breaks has led to neck and back discomfort that has required therapeutic attention to recover. Better to recognize your stress warning signals and practice self-care on the front end so that you can respond to needs as they come up and avoid the need for the two-by-four.

People have varying degrees of sensitivity when it comes to personal awareness. This can be a combination of nature and nurture. My husband and I fall on opposite ends of the spectrum of personal awareness. I am very sensitive. I'm aware of subtle changes in temperature. I notice when a hair falls down inside my shirt. I'm especially sensitive to toxins, like cigarette or cigar smoke or unnatural perfumes in public spaces. He jokingly has named a syndrome to describe my sensitivity. He calls it HABAS, or hyper-acute body awareness syndrome.

Steve, on the other end of the spectrum of sensitivity, is like a Labrador retriever—touch insensitive. Labs are bred to be able to run through brush and jump joyfully into icy, cold lakes to perform their job of retrieving a bird. Steve is similar in that he can go out into the yard to work, come in with a bloody hand, and not know how he injured himself. It just doesn't register. Some of this could be nature—like a hunting dog. But his medical education and professional training tend to demand and reinforce personal neglect at times.

Many careers occasionally require delayed gratification of needs. There are times when people can't acknowledge they are tired because they have three hours left on their shift. Or they ignore hunger pangs because they don't have time to eat. Our bodies are exquisite and very trainable. It is quite common to train the skill of ignoring personal needs in the service of work. Remember resilient to a fault?

I can't argue that this is all bad. It may be appropriate during stints of work that are busy. But it is a skill and can become a habit. And we all know how hard it is to change a habit. This incredible mind-body of yours can also be trained to recognize tipping points—when habits become harmful or when ignoring something can lead to injury. This skill is a necessary part of self-care.

Communication is a part of every healthy relationship. Nurturing the relationship with your whole self is part of good self-care. Your ability to thrive and even survive is dependent on tuning into communication holistically.

Awareness alerts you both to the tendencies that left unchecked contribute to disease AND the life-giving thoughts, choices, and behaviors that move you toward greater health. While it may be required to postpone self-care during a busy stretch at work, awareness informs you so you can plan self-care when you do have the time.

 Take a moment to reflect on the list of stress "signals" below. Notice that signals can show up in a variety of ways. Check off any that you recognize as familiar symptoms for you.

PHYSICAL SYMPTOMS

☐ Headaches   ☐ Sweaty palms   ☐ Tight neck

☐ Back Pain   ☐ Sleep issues   ☐ Restlessness

☐ Indigestion   ☐ Dizziness   ☐ Tiredness

☐ Stomachaches   ☐ Racing heart   ☐ Ringing in ears

BEHAVIORAL SYMPTOMS

☐ Excess smoking   ☐ Compulsive eating   ☐ Compulsive gum-chewing

☐ Bossiness

☐ Grinding of teeth   ☐ Attitude critical of others   ☐ Inability to get things done

☐ Overuse of alcohol

SPIRITUAL SYMPTOMS

- ☐ Emptiness
- ☐ Loss of meaning
- ☐ Doubt
- ☐ Unforgiving
- ☐ Cynicism
- ☐ Apathy
- ☐ Martyrdom
- ☐ Loss of direction

EMOTIONAL SYMPTOMS

- ☐ Crying
- ☐ Overwhelming pressure
- ☐ Anger
- ☐ Nervousness/ anxiety
- ☐ Loneliness
- ☐ Boredom-
- ☐ No meaning/ purpose
- ☐ Edginess
- ☐ Powerless to change
- ☐ Easily upset

COGNITIVE SYMPTOMS

- ☐ Trouble thinking clearly
- ☐ Lack of creativity
- ☐ Forgetfulness
- ☐ Constant worry
- ☐ Thoughts of running away
- ☐ No sense of humor

RELATIONAL SYMPTOMS

- ☐ Isolation
- ☐ Intolerance
- ☐ Resentment
- ☐ Lashing out
- ☐ Hiding
- ☐ Clamming up
- ☐ Nagging
- ☐ Lowered sex drive
- ☐ Distrust

Burnout

Unfortunately, the pace, intensity, and emotional vigilance required to sustain today's nonstop work culture are leading many to exhaustion or burnout. Work conditions aside (that would be another book!), poor body consciousness, mismanaged priorities, and lack of a clear wellness vision contribute to this epidemic condition. Hallmark components of burnout include: emotional exhaustion, reduced sense of personal accomplishment, and depersonalization.

Take a moment to check yourself for burnout by completing this self-test. Please note that this tool uses an informal approach to assessing burnout. It has not been validated through controlled scientific tests, and therefore, cannot be used as a diagnostic technique. For a rigorously validated test, refer to the Maslach Burnout Inventory.

Instructions

For each question, place a checkmark in the column that most applies to you. Add up your score and check your result using the scoring table underneath.

15 Statements to Answer					
Questions	Not at all = 1	Rarely =2	Sometime= 3	Often = 4	Very Often = 5
I feel run down and drained of physical or emotional energy.					
I have negative thoughts about my job.					
I am harder and less sympathetic with people than perhaps they deserve.					
I am easily irritated by small problems or by my coworkers and team.					
I feel misunderstood or unappreciated by my coworkers.					
I feel that I have no one to talk to.					
I feel that I am achieving less than I should.					

15 Statements to Answer					
Questions	Not at all = 1	Rarely =2	Sometime= 3	Often = 4	Very Often = 5
I feel an unpleasant level of pressure to succeed.					
I feel I am not getting what I want out of my job.					
I feel that I am in the wrong organization or the wrong profession.					
I am frustrated with parts of my job.					
I feel that organizational politics or bureaucracy frustrate my ability to do a good job.					
I feel that there is more to do than I practically have the ability to do.					
I feel that I do not have time to do many of the things that are important to doing a good quality job.					
I do not have time to plan as much as I would like to.					

Score interpretations (No matter your score, pay attention to areas you ranked a 5)

15-18: No sign of burnout.

19-32: Little sign of burnout.

33-49: At risk of burnout.

50-59: Severe risk of burnout.

60-75: Very severe risk of burnout.

(Adapted from MindTools.)[10]

Please consult your physician if you are concerned about the impact of stress on your health and well-being.

Stress is part of our human experience. Young adults struggle with the uncertainty of who they are and what their life path will look like. Others are distressed at the start of their careers and families as they chase the illustrious work/life balance. The mid-life working years are "sandwiched" with caring for children and aging parents. Others are afflicted by work culture or career changes, a growing sense of fatigue with the monotony of life and work, or some personal crisis.

If wellness is to be achieved throughout our lifespan, then you must be willing to shift self-care to a priority. You'll have to become astute about recognizing the presence and impact of stress in your life, both good and bad, and muster the courage to implement change.

---

[10] Mind Tools: Essential skills for excellent career. n.d. Burnout Self-Test. Accessed June 30, 2019. https://www.mindtools.com/pages/article/newTCS_08.htm.

Stop Takeaways

STOP. SHIFT HAPPENS.

This STOP section of the book is one you can revisit to refine, adapt, or change your life vision. Grounding yourself in self-care, growing in self-awareness, and aligning with your vision becomes a way of living.

- **Check in with your holistic well-being.**
- **Make self-care a priority.** Self-care generates the energy and mood to achieve your goals.
- **Have a clear vision.** Name it. Train it. Achieve it.
- **Know your stress warning signals.** Listen to your body and mind for holistic and sustainable living.
- **Look for and savor the equally true.**
- **SHIFT Happens.**

Breathe

The quieter you become,
the more you can hear.

—Ram Dass

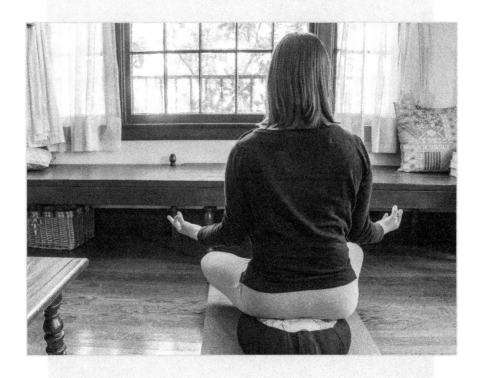

Chapter 5

Self-Regulation

Emotional Regulation and Resilience

Emotions are often overlooked during lifestyle change efforts. Goal setting can only take you so far. Effective and sustainable behavioral changes need to take into consideration how the emotional domain impacts and influences the change process. Emotions are energy. They can either derail or support your goals.

Low-grade, depleting emotions can significantly impact and influence your choices and behavior if they dominate the quality of your experience. This is often why so many people are frustrated by the inability to maintain the positive lifestyle changes they seek.

You can put a plan into place that is strategic and well designed, but if you are exposed to chronic stress conditions and have difficulty self-regulating draining emotions, you are at a significant disadvantage when it comes to following through with your intentions. Many rely heavily on their willpower to meet the physical and emotional demands of their workday but lose that self-control when it comes to self-care.

Consider the content of your day. How often do you feel:

- ☐ Frustration – things not going your way, constant interruption, or distraction.

- ☐ Disappointment – requests, suggestions, ideas rejected, or denied.

- ☐ Devastation – personal or family problems or health issues that change the landscape and experience of your life.

- ☐ Impatience – the daily commute, being put on hold, attending ineffectual meetings, difficult relationships.

- ☐ Vigilance – being watchful of disruptive behavior, people, or events.

- ☐ Overwhelm – too much to do … too little time.

With the complexity of life today, our energy is under constant siege, making self-regulation of our emotions a necessary skill set for performance and sustainability.

Coherence: A Simple Overview

"Coherence" describes a state in which the heart, mind, and emotions are aligned and in sync. Physiologically, the immune, hormonal, and nervous systems function in a state of energetic coordination. The ability to alter one's emotional responses is central to energy regulation. This ability to self-regulate the feelings and emotions in response to moment-to-moment experiences is intimately tied to our physiology, exemplifying the intimate relationship of the body, mind, and emotional systems.[11]

---

[11] McCraty, Rollin, and Robert, R. Rees. 2009. "The Central Role of the Heart in Generating and Sustaining Positive Emotions." In *The Oxford Handbook of Positive Psychology,* by Shane, J. and Synder, C.R. Lopez, 527-536. New York: Oxford University Press.

Coherence is different than relaxation. Herbert Benson is an American medical doctor, cardiologist, and founder of the Mind/ Body Medical Institute at Massachusetts General Hospital (MGH) in Boston. He pioneered mind/body medicine as support for health and healing. His book, *The Relaxation Response*, describes that it is within our conscious control to reverse the effects of the stress response back to a restful state. Relaxation has been scientifically proven to be an effective treatment for a wide range of stress-related disorders. In fact, to the extent that any disease is caused or made worse by stress, downregulation of the stress response can help.[12]

Deep relaxation is not always a feasible option during the course of a hectic day. I've been teaching yoga, guided relaxation/imagery, and other relaxation strategies for a long time. And while I still promote these practices, many of my clients are reluctant to participate because of time constraints and the belief that relaxing midday would just make returning to work more difficult. Relaxation, then, is postponed for when they are free to relax … and that seemed to never happen due to competing priorities.

Unlike deep relaxation, coherence is an alert but balanced state that helps protect your energy during the course of hectic days. This state is preferable when excess energy drain is problematic, but deeper relaxation may not be appropriate. It only takes a few minutes, and all you need is your breath and awareness. You don't need a gym or yoga class. You can achieve this state in your office, in a meeting, or during a stressful commute.

Consider the role of the heart. Coherence is the "sweet spot" for energy regulation, and the key lies with the heart. For our entire lifespan, the heart pumps blood, supplying the brain and body with the oxygen and nutrients we require for survival. Without our heart beating, we cannot live. The heart is only able to sustain this work

---

[12]   Benson, H. 1975. *The Relaxation Response*. New York: William Morrow.

by prioritizing self-care. The heart nourishes itself *FIRST* with blood flow through the coronary arteries. If that self-care is interrupted or blocked, we suffer a heart attack and potentially die as a result. Self-care is NEVER a selfish act. It is an essential resilience strategy that needs to be sustained throughout our lifespan.

> The heart doesn't take care of itself just on the weekends, vacation, or day off. Self-care is integral to every action, to every beat of the heart.

The heart is also widely recognized as the anatomical location for our emotions. We are "heartbroken" when we are sad. Almost without thinking, we put our hand at our heart when we experience wonder or awe. We even pat our chest to demonstrate the acceleration of our heart with excitement. An athlete has a lot of "heart" when passionate about competition. We place a hand over our hearts when we pledge allegiance to our flag. And many traditions draw hands to the heart in prayer. And of course, the red heart shape is the iconic symbol of romantic love. The powerful impact of emotions and the role of the heart is not "woo woo." This is science.

The heart and our emotions play an essential role in self-regulation and resilience. We would like to think that our cognition and intellect can plan, prioritize, strategize, and execute our way to health and well-being. But the evidence is clear ...

> *Emotions often drive or derail our decision-making and behaviors.*

The Heart-Brain connection. Emotions affect the neural activity of the heart. The heart sends this information to the brain via the autonomic nervous system and influences the brain centers associated with thinking, decision-making, reaction times, long- and short-term memory, and self-regulation.[13] The thalamus, a key brain center, is involved in optimal function and is strongly affected by neural signals from the heart.

One of the many roles of the thalamus is to synchronize the neural activity of the entire brain, including the cortex, which is the thinking part of the brain. The cortex is where executive functions take place: the ability to plan and set goals, think abstractly and creatively, self-regulate, and forecast how actions and behaviors will affect the future. Are you beginning to see why influencing these functions may serve you well?

Coherence is achieved through two things:

- Simple breath regulation *and*
- Connecting to a steady flow of restorative emotions

While Benson's work describes the physiological relationship of stress to several body systems (heart rate, breathing, muscle tension, blood pressure, and metabolism), coherence uses heart rate variability as an indicator of the fascinating relationship between emotions, the heart, and the brain.[14] Coherence is an effective target for self-regulation skills to support optimal mood, energy, clear thinking, and resilience.

Achieving coherence is easier than people expect. I use heart rhythm coherence feedback to support skill development. But even without

---

[13] McCraty, Rollin, and Robert, R. Rees. 2009. "The Central Role of the Heart in Generating and Sustaining Positive Emotions." In *The Oxford Handbook of Positive Psychology,* by Shane, J. and Synder, C.R. Lopez, 527-536. New York: Oxford University Press.

[14] McCraty, Rollin, and Robert, R. Rees. 2009. "The Central Role of the Heart in Generating and Sustaining Positive Emotions." In *The Oxford Handbook of Positive Psychology,* by Shane, J. and Synder, C.R. Lopez, 527-536. New York: Oxford University Press.

equipment for feedback, you can train yourself to balance your breath and direct the quality of your inner experience. Choosing restorative emotions preserves and promotes energy, while draining emotions maintain heavy, dragging, or upsetting feelings. The challenge lies in convincing yourself that this alert and balanced state feels better, produces more, and is far more sustainable than the accelerated pace and sometimes chaotic experience of busy days.

Heart rate variability is not the same as heart rate. It is the beat-to-beat variation of the rate of the heart, which is influenced by breath and emotion. It can be captured, plotted, and reflected as a sine wave that is called a heart rhythm pattern.

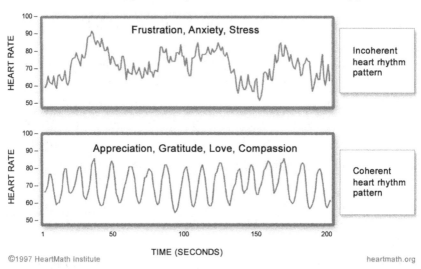

Fig. 1 Emotions are reflected in heart rhythm patterns. The heart rhythm pattern shown in the top graph, characterized by an erratic, irregular pattern (incoherence), is typical of draining emotions such as anger or frustration. The example in the bottom graph shows a coherent heart rhythm pattern, typically observed when an individual is experiencing sustained, restorative emotions.

Incoherent heart rhythms, triggered by draining emotions, interfere with the brain's ability to synchronize cortical activity, causing what scientists call cortical inhibition.

While not always comfortable, the full range of human emotion serves a purpose in the appropriate context. Thus, we avoid labeling any emotion as good or bad.

On the other hand, coherent heart rhythms generated by balanced breathing and restorative emotions (like peace, gratitude, or care) can improve what scientists call cortical facilitation. **Cortical facilitation** means all of the executive functions are optimized. In other words, when we're coherent, we can make appropriate choices, improve reaction times, access memory, and enhance focus, creativity, and the ability to problem-solve.

This physiologic interplay becomes relevant to our self-care when a draining emotion hijacks our attention and mindlessly engages us in drama that disconnects us from our self-care goals or right living. Impatience, irritability, and other draining emotions can lead us to do stupid things. Sometimes we even say, "What was I thinking?" Often, we weren't thinking! The cortex was inhibited. We literally can't think expansively when we feel stressed or tethered to an emotional storyline … whether real or imagined.

Incoherence sometimes leads to "thoughtless" reactions. Have you ever been upset and reacted to someone with words or actions you later regretted? When this happens, has it typically lead to more stress and wasted time? How many times have you done this with the same person? In response to the same issue? For example, perhaps you've repeatedly asked your teenager to clean their room, only to find it's still a disaster after your 10-hour day at work. Frustration leads you to an emotional outburst … and, to top it off, their comeback is, "What's your problem?" This can escalate into an argument that continues to drain energy.

All of our human emotions serve an important purpose at the appropriate time. Consider the scenario with a mother chasing after her child who is running into traffic. Fear of the impending danger creates a cascade of biologic changes described as the stress response. Cortisol, a stress hormone, floods the body, along with hundreds of other neurochemicals, facilitating her ability to get to her child, swiftly pick her up, and safely return her to the house. Once the threat is over, it takes time to recover. Cortisol is processed slowly in the body and can have lasting effects on mood and energy.

When you experience a positive emotion and are energetically balanced or coherent, your body has another hormone, DHEA or the "vitality hormone," which also generates a cascade of reactions. Conversely, this physiologic state supports greater mental and emotional flexibility and composure. No yoga mat needed. And with training, you can achieve this high-performance state within a few minutes. This built-in pharmacopeia of sorts is at our disposal to use with skill and intention. By training our mind-body awareness and executing discipline in self-regulation, we can become skilled in generating the internal environment that facilitates appropriate and effective engagement with life, relationships, and work.

 ## Working the Concept of "Equally True"

I introduced the idea of "equally true" in an earlier section. This concept plays an important role when shifting into coherence. My adult daughter came to me with an issue that had her emotionally upset. Instead of addressing the problem with her, we did an exercise to shift her mood. I coached her to bring balance to her breath and invited her to cultivate imagery of a scene that brings her a sense of peace and contentment. Emotional regulation doesn't have to look like a yoga class. No incense or lotus pose required.

I let her linger with her breath and imagery for about a minute and then simply asked her to bring her issue to mind. Then I asked, "From this vantage point, did your perspective of your problem change? " Her eyes had been closed for her visualization. She opened her eyes with a smile and said, "That's cheating!"

She had just experienced the power of reclaiming her inner quality of peace from the snare of negativity that limits thinking. From this inner quality of peace, generated by thoughts that are "equally true," several things happened. Her perspective changed, for sure. The problem was no longer so overwhelming. And as she generated restorative emotion, her capacity for creativity improved, and several possible remedies emerged. All this took less than five minutes to experience and process. Consider the physical toll of lingering stress she was able to avoid.

Her comment that this approach was "cheating" is interesting. Why do we sometimes think that problem-solving has to be difficult and uncomfortable? Why does hard work have to be so hard? Consider the amount of energy you could save by freeing yourself from depleting emotions that often accompany even simple problems and allowing yourself to explore the possibility of a positive mind.

Learning to sustain coherence or the inner quality of peace quickly brings more stability to your system. From this inner landscape, you can more readily identify a path of action that aligns with your values and purpose.

This is especially relevant and important for those in careers where a stress response accompanies most daily work experiences, including fields like police, fire, military, healthcare, and others. These individuals are highly trained to function effectively under stressful conditions. However, it is possible to experience the stress response *and* maintain coherence at the same time. It may take repetition and training to learn to stabilize emotions within stressful scenarios, but it's possible (and often necessary).

Equally important is competence at downregulating to restore the body and mind after taxing episodes of stress. The inability to downregulate after stressful events and restore coherence comes at a cost to the human system, increasing the risk of emotional instability, sleep disruption, fatigue, and burnout. Achieving coherence and relaxation can be difficult if we support energy and mood with caffeine or sugar. This can make downregulation that much more difficult.

Mastery over emotional regulation requires a holistic approach, which means attention to what we consume in food, beverages, and even entertainment. The quantity and quality of sleep is another important consideration. A holistic wellness plan considers the role that each dimension of your well-being contributes to nurturing an inner quality of peace or coherence.

Using heart rhythm monitoring to obtain feedback on mind-body interventions can help train and sustain coherence for positive transformation. Maurita, an emergency department nurse, relied on this technique to improve her self-regulation practices, which assisted her in the midst of challenging personal circumstances.

She has aging parents with health issues and is a single parent with two sons, one with substance abuse issues. Her work in a level one trauma emergency department can be grueling and emotionally challenging. She came to me to relieve the stress that was "roaring" within her, which was disrupting her sleep, relationships, and workflow.

She practiced the Mindful Pause with the aid of heart rhythm monitoring to measure her coherence. She also began practicing a variety of mind-body skills to support self-regulation. Within one month, her ability to self-regulate her heart rhythm pattern into coherence improved significantly. The images below show the pattern at the start of our work and one month later. You don't need to understand heart rate variability to see the shift from a chaotic and imbalanced rhythm to one that is smooth and balanced.

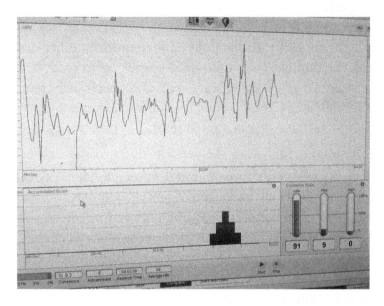

March 4, 2019 – 91% low coherence

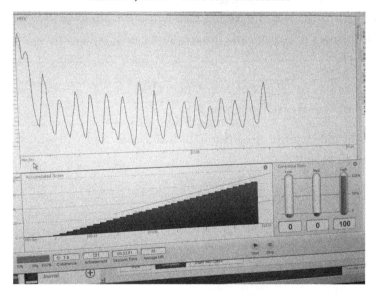

April 5, 2019 – 100% High Coherence

Her April session is particularly amazing. It occurred four days after she had taken a day off of work due to the overwhelm caused by stress. Her adult son, who struggles with addiction, had broken into her apartment and stolen some things. In the aftermath of this event, she needed a personal day to deal with the police and coordinate other details. At the time, she thought she would need a week off to recover. Instead, she practiced her growing self-care skills and, remarkably, returned to work after only one day off. When she came to her appointment at the end of the week, she demonstrated masterful proficiency in eliciting coherence.

Both sessions were only three minutes in length. Her self-regulation proficiency came from a variety of simple self-care practices that take very little time out of the day and require just a little practice to master. Once clients are familiar with the sensation of coherence, they intuitively gravitate to practices that work well for them, sometimes discovering that they have practices of their own that they simply lost track of over time. In this case, it was a combination of the Mindful Pause, a Three Blessings Exercise, and a hot shower with uplifting music! All of these self-care choices worked to help shift breath and mood in order to restore the inner quality of stability and peace … or coherence.

For a complete overview of coherence, visit: HeartMath.org/Research/Science-of-the-Heart/Coherence/

Next, we will explore how the Mindful Pause tool can support your skill development.

Chapter 6

Mindful Pause – Tool for Self-Regulation

Our minds can become clogged with the busyness and details of living – things that make us fret and squirm, things that make us run from waiting and the slow greening of our soul. That's when we need to pause ...

–Sue Monk Kidd

Whether it's having a difficult conversation with a supervisor, executing a complex skill under stressful conditions, parenting an upset child, or witnessing a loved one pass, we all know the events in life that make us fret and squirm. Training inner stability with Mindful Pause opens us to being changed, touched, moved, inspired, and ultimately transformed by the very experiences we might choose to avoid.

Your MAP is your vision. The Stop, Breathe, Think, Choose process interrupts the auto-pilot pattern that often accompanies busy and complex lives and trains the self-regulation that leads to personal growth and transformation. The Mindful Pause tool is the means to make your vision your reality.

Mindful Pause for Meditation is a formal practice that trains a new baseline of stability and peace in a controlled setting, making it easier to access the trained mindfulness state when meeting challenges.

Mindful Pause for Mindfulness serves as an on-the-go tool to increase present moment awareness, reduce reactivity, and better regulate mood and energy with intentional living in the rhythm of life.

Growing Your Meaning & Purpose

When you live into the Mindful Pause to stop, breath, think, and choose, you accept an invitation to interrupt living a life dictated by external pressures, cultural expectations, or habits. It fosters self-awareness and grows the capacity to live in a way aligned with your core values, personal faith, or life philosophy. This enriches the meaning and purpose domain of your well-being.

Deepening your sense of meaning and purpose enriches intentional living and connects you with the "why" of your lifestyle choices so that "I should" turns into "I want." What you eat and how you move, sleep, work, play, cope, and relate to others can all be enriched by deepening your sense of meaning and purpose.

Dozens of studies repeatedly demonstrate that people who believe their lives have meaning or purpose appear to be better off. For example, they are happier and profess greater overall well-being, life satisfaction, control over their lives, and feel more engaged in work. They also report fewer adverse effects, such as depression and anxiety, workaholism, suicidal ideation, and substance abuse, and they have less need for therapy.[15]

---

[15] Steger, Michael F. 2009. "Meaning in Life." In *The Oxford Handbook of Positive Psychology,* by Shane, J. Lopez and C.R. Snyder, 679-687. New York: Oxford University Press.

The Mindful Pause can begin a diverse and rewarding journey toward discovering or rediscovering your meaning and purpose. Given competing commitments, you may have a life philosophy or faith that from which you're disconnected. Or, you may be beginning a journey toward noticing and naming the virtues or beliefs that drive your commitments, preferences, and actions. No matter where you find yourself, a personal practice is essential for self-regulation development and growing a satisfying life by deepening your sense of meaning and purpose. Toward that end, I encourage you to consider creating your own sacred space to nurture your self-care practice.

Create Your Sacred Space

Creating sacred space supports an intention to connect deeply with yourself and each moment with a quality of sacredness or devotion. I suggest choosing a space or place as special and designating it as the location where you go to focus on personal growth. Fundamental to your self-care plan is time dedicated to meditation, inspiration, relaxation, and personal reflection. The purpose of this time is to grow the self-regulation and spiritual muscles required for holistic living. This is hallowed work. These practices will take greater root when cultivated in a restorative place, unplugged from your demanding, perhaps messy, and overly full life.

Many dismiss this step as arbitrary or of little relevance. But you will come to recognize the value of creating your own oasis. All kinds of spaces are designed to support function and purpose. Your workspace is likely designed to support organization and efficiency. Garages, kitchens, and stores are all intentionally designed to serve a particular purpose.

There's something powerful in physically stepping into a space that has the intended purpose of self-care. You may already have this reaction to certain places. You may have a place—a vacation home, a spot on a familiar walk, or your church or temple—that just by stepping into it, you experience ease or peace. Consider how you can recreate that feeling in your own home.

Choose a place that you can design for comfort and inspiration. Perhaps you have a favorite chair or spot by a window where you can train your body and mind to sink into a more present frame of mind just by entering the space. You don't need a lot of room, but the area should be clear of clutter and away from visual reminders of other obligations or distractions, like your work, household clutter, family members, phone, TV, or computer. It also helps to have a simple item of beauty like a candle, flower, stone, or shell—any meaningful or sacred image that connects you to a restorative feeling of peace, contentment, beauty, devotion, or love.

Here is a picture of my sacred space. The candle reminds me of the presence of the Divine in my midst. The word "Peace" connects me to my personal practice of praying St. Francis' Prayer for Peace. I usually have an inspirational book there to support my desire for wisdom from a variety of voices. And you see my meditation stool and cushion. You will read more about that in a bit.

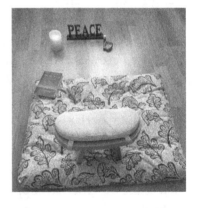

You may want to let the people in your life know that when you enter this space, you are not to be interrupted, demonstrating the value that self-care and unplugging are important aspects of living well. I had one client who wore a sound elimination headset. She let her family know that when they saw her with that headset on, she was not to be interrupted. She also needed to quiet the sound triggers that would pull her back into engagement with competing priorities, like the buzz of the dryer alarm, the ping of a text message coming in, or the bark of the dog as someone approaches the house. You get the idea.

> For as complex and draining as our lives can become, everyone should have access to a sacred space on a daily basis ... right in their home.

You may find that you have a couple of spaces where you can retreat, depending on your intention or even the weather. Here in Minnesota, where I do most of my work, our winters are long. When weather permits, clients often benefit from intentionally designing a self-care spot on their patio, screened porch (the mosquito is often claimed as our state bird), or in their yard. For some of my clients who have a significant commute, the car becomes their sacred space. They take a brief Mindful Pause there before or after their commute to generate the mood and energy for appropriate self-care.

 # Mindfulness and Meditation

Mindfulness

Nowadays, meditation and mindfulness are often used interchangeably, which can be confusing. I consider mindfulness, for the purpose of my coaching, to be a state of awareness that you develop in the formal practice of meditation, and you then learn to access in the course of daily life. Mindfulness, by Jon Kabat Zinn's definition, describes this state as "paying attention in a particular way, on purpose, in the present moment and non-judgmentally"[16] I consider meditation the formal practice of growing this skill.

---

[16]   Kabat-Zinn, Jon. 1990. *Full Catastrophe Living: using the wisdom of your body and mind to face stress, pain, and illness.* New York: Delcorte Press.

Given that mindfulness is an important target for personal growth and development, it is important to understand early on what mindfulness is NOT:

- Relaxation
- A religion—though it can be part of a religious practice
- A way to change thoughts
- Difficult or easy
- A way not to be concerned with the future anymore
- Impossible to investigate scientifically

Relaxation is a worthy, but different intention. Benson's "relaxation response" describes an important state of being that allows the body to self-heal and replenish itself. The unrelenting pace and task loading of days, however, is not always conducive to downregulating all the way to relaxation.

Once habituated to high-pace living, many are not willing to interrupt their pace with relaxation for fear that they won't be able to ramp it up again to re-engage with work. This attitude is captured in the familiar saying, "keep your nose to the grindstone." While mindfulness in its purest sense is not relaxation, it likely will feel like relaxation given the amplified state of "busy-ness" that so many have grown accustomed to as normal.

If restful sleep is your goal, the Mindful Pause *can* be a gateway to deeper relaxation or part of a sleep hygiene practice. *Intention is a central aspect of any practice.* Be clear about what you want to accomplish.

Mindfulness is not a religion, but it can support spirituality. One can study more deeply the meditative traditions from any one of the five religions of the world—Christianity, Buddhism, Judaism, Hinduism, or Islam. If you have a religious orientation, I encourage you to consider the wisdom there as inspiration and support for growing your practice and deepening your sense of Meaning and Purpose. Spirituality, or your path to deeper ways of knowing self in relationship to self, others, the world, and the Divine, is a deeply personal journey and can span a lifetime. Living in alignment with your spirit or purpose inspires meaning that most find deeply satisfying.

Mindfulness is not a way to change your thoughts. As a coach, people come to visit with me at times in their life when their thoughts and emotions are disruptive. Sometimes, people hope that like ibuprofen lessens pain, meditation will help them lessen their current suffering. In some ways, it does, but not by changing, resisting, or denying thoughts, rather by allowing them to appear and pass without judgment, control, or clinging. Difficult emotions do not last forever. By anchoring awareness on the breath and the sensation of noticing and allowing what is, you can grow and sustain peace.

Mindfulness is simple in its instruction ... but not easy. It takes practice and repetition to develop the skill to become mindful, but then you get to benefit from the fruits of your labor. This is why I introduce the use of Mindful Pause as both meditation practice and as a tool for in-the-moment self-regulation. Formal practice trains the body-mind connection so that stability and peace are more easily accessed on-the-go to meet our daily challenges.

Mindfulness does not free us from being engaged with the future. There is a role, time, and place for applying the gifts of our cognitive capacity to envision, plan, forecast, and strategize. The Mindful Pause allows you to access and savor the wisdom of the present moment, connecting you to peace to align with your authentic self, so you can engage in the world and move into the future with confidence, clarity, and purpose.

Mindfulness is not impossible to investigate scientifically. In addition to the centuries of effort from the wisdom traditions, science is now contributing a deeper understanding of the many "fruits" of meditation, mindfulness, prayer, and other spiritual practices, making access to benefits available from a variety of sources. Science has explored love, gratitude, compassion, empathy, meditation, altruism, and prayer and contributed a deeper understanding and validation of spiritual practices to health and well-being.[17] Mindfulness, in particular, has become a popular topic within the field of scientific research, with the number of publications dedicated to the topic rising significantly over recent years.

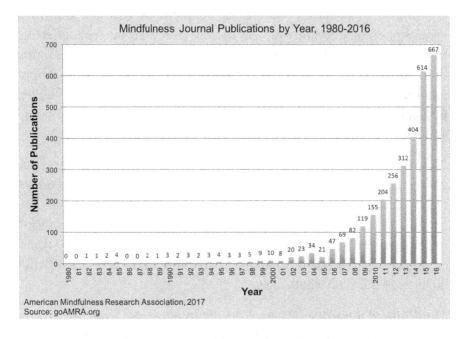

Mindfulness journal publications by year, 1980-2018.[18]

---

[17] Pargament, Kenneth I, and Annette Mahoney. 2009. "Spirituality: The Search for the Sacred." In *The Oxford Handbook of Positive Psychology*, by Shane J Lopez and C.R. Snyder, 611-619. New York: Oxford University Press.

[18] American Mindfulness Research Association. 2019. Resources. Accessed June 30, 2019. www.goamra.org

Meditation

Formal practice occurs in your Sacred Space. The Mindful Pause is an effective practice for beginners seeking to grow a meditation practice that supports mindfulness. I like to refer to meditation as your chosen *formal practice,* which finds you practicing in a quiet, undistracted space.

This helps you to experience a deep peace and connection of self with the Divine or the "something larger than self." You learn to refine the skill of self-regulation and sustain this deeper connection, resulting in the development of a body, mind, spirit connection that can be more easily tapped during life's challenging times to support self-regulation.

Formal meditation practice has many paths. Centering prayer, yoga, Transcendental Meditation, chanting, mantra meditation, and Mindfulness-Based Stress Reduction are a few of these paths. The Spiritual muscles that grow in these practices (detachment, peace, love, kindness, gratitude, compassion, perseverance, forgiveness, etc.) become the armor that defends against assault from an unpredictable and challenging world.

Usually, a Mindful Pause in the moment helps to discern the method or practice that suits a particular season or moment of life. By experimentation, you can continually adapt and modify your practice to fit your situation and needs. Flexibility in your practice gives you a range of practices to apply in a variety of situations.

Traditionally, meditation is a practice of stillness. But movement practices can be a gateway into stillness and can serve as teachers for the difficult transition that we all seek in choosing to stop. Yoga, Qigong, Tai Chi are disciplines that improve or develop inner stability combined with a physical challenge. They offer the means to train awareness of tension and cultivate discernment, self-regulation, and higher consciousness.

I encourage movement practices for those who find it difficult to practice sitting meditation ... or stillness of any kind. The exertion of the physical body, connected with the breath, provides a sensation that serves as an anchor for attention. Feeling, moving, and breathing releases energy that helps prepare you to experience the continued growth that can be experienced in stillness.

Others may prefer a more pure approach, choosing a particular method and diving deep into that one practice for personal growth. I have done this at times to experience one method or another more deeply. Each year, for example, I spend at least five days in silent retreat, guided by the Mindfulness-Based Stress Reduction (MBSR) method. Or I participate in a retreat or conference around spirituality or meditation. This always deepens my practice and sets a course for another year of personal growth.

I have studied Ignatian and Benedictine spirituality, Christian Centering Prayer, Buddhism, and Yoga. Additionally, I've trained in Jon Kabat Zinn's Mindfulness-Based Stress Reduction (MBSR). I have read the inspirations of great spiritual teachers like Cynthia Bourgeault, Thich Nhat Hanh, Pema Chodron, and others. I've studied the psychophysiology work from the HeartMath Institute and experts like Dr. Richard Davidson of the Center for Healthy Minds, and Dr. Daniel Siegel of the UCLA Mindful Awareness Research Center. By reading a variety of voices from different perspectives, I feel confident encouraging clients to explore a variety of voices as well. Wisdom is abundant.

Over the years, I've been especially drawn to voices that integrate science, spirituality, and religion. I often recommend Roger Walsh's book, *Essential Spirituality*, to those who are curious about spiritual growth but want to explore practices from a variety of wisdom traditions. Jon Kabat Zinn's work is renowned for taking traditional Buddhist practices and delivering them with a secular voice into western medicine. And it was especially important and very formative for me to discover the work of Thomas Ryan, a Paulist priest and certified yoga teacher, to encourage my understanding of the body as sacred and our temple for spiritual growth.

Mindful Pause is not intended to be a comprehensive analysis of the world religions nor a prescription for adopting mine. Instead, it is an introductory approach intended to help you discern your own.

I invite you into the laboratory of your own body and mind to experiment with meditation and mindfulness as a strategy to wake up to the present moment, train the observer mind, and transform the way you experience the world and your life experiences by leading from your source and strengths.

Meditation trains the mind-body connection. Perhaps you have used practice and repetition to learn another skill. Formal practice, of any form, is a skill that requires consistency and determination. Think of it as equivalent to training your body repetitively for job proficiency, athletic skill, or going to a quiet library to study a chosen subject. You are training a strong mind-body connection to generate and sustain stability and peace.

Formal practice explores anchored attention and the gift of non-doing. Practice best occurs in a controlled setting to rehearse and memorize the mind-body skills of:

- Non-doing
- Anchored attention
- Body awareness
- Surrender to the reality of each moment

Whether you are in your sacred space, a church or temple, or outside in the temple of the woods, you simply need dedicated time to practice.

Back in high school, my free throw percentage was very high. I developed this skill through a lot of practice. In addition to any free throws that were built into our regular practice, I would go into a quiet gym, usually by myself, and I would shoot 25 free throws at every hoop. There were 6. Step to the line … take three dribbles … spin the ball to rest in my right hand … feel the grain of the ball and the seam at my fingertips. Breathe … then I'd smoothly hinge at my ankles, knees, and hips, sensing into my entire body, from my feet to the crown of my head. With a coordinated lift, I would track my elbow, arm, wrist, and fingers through a memorized path that ended with the "gooseneck" wrist of every good shooter and the sound of the swish as the ball passed through the net. Repeat.

Learning how to drive, play a musical instrument, or any particular job skill requires repetition and practice to train the muscle memory of the brain-body connection. Our bodies and minds are complex and amazing. You can train your body, mind, and spirit to be your ally and coach. I won't attempt to take you on a deep dive into either the spiritual or scientific exploration. I leave that journey to you.

Chapter 7

Mindful Pause
for Meditation

The Mindful Pause is meant to be a tool for meditation and mindfulness. The Mindful Pause serves most beginners well and can be a gateway into deeper study. It also serves as a practical way to restore the body, mind, and spirit. It draws from several sources I've found on my personal quest—spiritual and religious traditions, meditation teachers, and empirical evidence. Clients and retreatants of mine have found this approach to be easily accessible, approachable, and adaptable to their personal preferences. One client shared:

Cami has a very down to earth approach to mindfulness practice, which is important for introducing people to these practices without coming across as dogmatic.

– Psychiatry resident, workshop participant

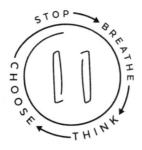

The Mindful Pause is an introduction to mindful living that can be easily integrated into busy lifestyles. The steps of stopping, breathing, and being in the body—sustaining the awareness of inner peace and stability and choosing to act in alignment with your MAP—sustains your journey. The circular depiction of the Mindful Pause intentions (stop, breathe, think, choose) reflects the dynamic flow and evolution of this practice.

The target for meditation is a calm but alert state, and the intentions of the Mindful Pause guide you there with simplicity and ease. Downregulation of the busy mind and body can be challenging when slowing down is most strongly connected to sleep—since that's about the only time that most people "settle down." Therefore, a seated posture with a long spine supports the effort to stay awake during your practice.

 ## Posture is Fundamental to Meditation Practice.

Postures have meaning. Assuming a posture that embodies the intentions that we seek engages the body, mind, and spirit for restoration. I suggest a seated mountain pose with a long spine tall to the crown of your head. Becoming a "mountain" invites the qualities of stability, resilience, dignity, and beauty to accompany your practice of peace.

Mountain posture allows the breath to move easily through the body. Imagine what happens when there is a kink in a hose when watering a garden. The flow of water stops! So, too, when we lose our dignified upright posture, the full range of motion of the breath is stopped. Life and inspiration are in the breath. You can experiment with a variety of postures that afford you comfort but also keep you awake, with access to the full range of motion of your breath. Posture provides full access to the breath. And the breath gives access to peace.

Retire the No Pain, No Gain Approach

The traditional posture is seated cross-legged on the floor or meditation cushion. Proper alignment is achieved when your knees rest below your hips. This alignment is nearly impossible for most Americans since we have very tight hips! Early in my meditation training, I attempted to sit like a "yogi." I propped myself up on a meditation cushion to elevate my hips, crossed my legs, and envisioned myself a budding saint. What I experienced was far from holy! The posture left me with tightness and discomfort in my knees, ankles, hips, low back, and shoulders.

My self-talk was even worse. I criticized and complained about all the ways I failed at meditation. My habituated "no pain, no gain" approach did not help either! "Come on, Cam, you can make it another 10 minutes! Suck it up!" Punishing myself by training in an uncomfortable posture completely defeats the purpose of meditation ... to embody and memorize a stable, peaceful, and alert awareness. Meditation is not about forcing or enduring. It's about allowing and maintaining a sense of peace and lightness of being. Keeping this in mind transforms the "no pain, no gain" approach into the "know pain, know gain" stance. When you establish a stable foundation, you engage in the practice of knowing yourself.

I spent two painful days of trying to meditate seated cross-legged on the floor studying with a yogi at an ashram in India. Noticing my discomfort, he offered this advice, "many saints have come to enlightenment sitting in a chair." I could have kissed him! Since then, I let go of my attachment to one way of meditating and have experimented with many postures for my practice.

Attending a Mindfulness Based Stress Reduction seven-day silent retreat in Colorado, I was pleased to be introduced to a "prayer stool." It allows you to sit comfortably in a kneeling posture, knees below the hips while maintaining a long spine. I was amazed that I could sit easily for 45 minutes without an aching back, stiff hips, or painful knees—and stay awake! As a cradle Catholic, I had to chuckle to myself that, of course, I would be most comfortable on my knees!

Eyes Open or Closed?

Some people find it difficult to meditate with eyes closed since that "posture" is so strongly associated with sleep. The upright mountain posture may help. But if you find that it is difficult to stay alert, you can experiment with your eyes open with a soft, downward gaze, perhaps focusing on an item of beauty, like a candle, flower, or spiritual icon. There is much variation between individuals on the ability to sustain attention.

For some, eyes closed gives the "monkey mind" a free pass, and all the "monkeys" go wild, creating and following distractions. These people may find that with eyes open, they have better control of the "monkey mind" by having a visual target to keep their brain occupied. Feel free to experiment with what works best for you.

If you choose to practice with eyes closed, direct your inner gaze at a point above and between the eyes. Even with eyes closed, it is possible to *look away*. In a lengthy sit, when my mind wanders off from my present moment awareness, I notice that my inner gaze shifts as well. My gaze can wander from the *focused* and *present* feeling that comes with the mind narrowed to my brow to lifting up and off to the right or left as if I am "looking" at my distraction. When I notice, I simply return, without judgment or harsh criticism, to my next breath.

Practice Non-Doing

As I established earlier, our culture is addicted to our "doingness." We are important, relevant, and productive when we are "doing" something—usually working. Many have lost the wisdom that non-doing or "beingness" is an essential restorative practice. And the "quality" of our doingness is often burdened with a sense of overwhelm.

Sleep is the most commonly practiced non-doing activity. The accelerated nature of most days, however, and poor self-regulation skills, sometimes makes sleep less than satisfying. Some even continue their work through their dreams!

Beyond the necessity for the body to restore itself, the wakeful state of non-doing trains the body-mind to be comfortable with stillness and to practice steadiness and anchored attention through the experience of distraction. Why is this important? Because the incessant nature of our "doingness," where we are often attempting to engage with multiple tasks at the same time, is what contributes to fatigue, burnout, and dis-ease. Strengthening the muscle of attention and remaining steady can improve performance at work and satisfaction with rest.

Working with the Busy Mind

Too many people believe that meditation is just not for them. Their minds are "too busy," they "never stop," and they "can't remain still" for any period of time. This feeling is not unique. Most of humanity is challenged by an easily distracted mind. The mind is designed to be busy, and the body follows. People fidget, squirm, rock, tap, hum, or whistle to avoid stillness. There are great treasures to be discovered in stillness.

When we start in the body and assume a posture of stillness, we can begin to work on the skill of narrowing our focus and training the mind to follow the body. Everyone struggles with attention. And everyone can also benefit from training this skill. It is a skill that can transform your life, work, and relationships. Whether people are born to be wired or they've conditioned themselves to constant "busyness," the evidence overwhelmingly supports the benefit of practicing "non-doing" for restoration and sustaining present moment awareness for mindful attention.

Applying the skill of a trained narrow focus improves safety, productivity, and satisfaction at work. In relationships, you become less reactionary and better able to listen and respond in healthy ways. Life seems less hurried and more rich and meaningful when you allow yourself to experience it one moment at a time. And ultimately, the quality of presence that the Mindful Pause helps you touch is the alignment we seek to live into our best life.

Now we can explore the Mindful Pause as self-care practice to grow present moment awareness and self-regulation.

Stop

Many of us have been running all our lives. Practice stopping.

–Thich Nhat Hanh

Stopping and intentionally setting aside time for deliberate practice is an act of self-care. Stopping for stillness honors the natural rhythm between doing and being. Both are essential manifestations of our human experience. The non-doing aspect of our experience of vital living is greatly underappreciated. We never let the dust settle before chasing the next task.

With Mindful Pause presence, we come to trust that work actually continues in our non-doing or "beingness." Our body, mind, and spirit need stillness to integrate our experiences, restore harmony to body systems, and surrender our attachments and distractions to create the spaciousness for virtue, meaning, and purpose to emerge and grow.

You honor the need to stop when you:

- Enter your sacred space.
- Commit to a regular and disciplined mindfulness or devotional practice.
- Assume a dignified posture.
- Breathe and sustain inner peace and stability.
- Let go of expectation.
- Establish the inner qualities that inspire your outward living.

Breathe

Breath is medicine. Diaphragmatic breathing or full-range-of-motion breathing has significant benefits to our body and mind and is an essential element of most meditative and spiritual traditions as well. The benefits include physiologic changes, emotional regulation, and spiritual transformation.

Physiologic changes:

- Restores balance to the autonomic nervous system
- Activates the immune system
- Decreases blood pressure
- Releases physical and emotional tension
- Improves flow of blood and lymph
- Improves digestion[19]

---

[19] Rakel, David. 2007. "Integrative Medicine." In *Guided Imagery and Interactive Guided Imagery,* by MD Martin L. Rossman, 1031-1037. Philadelphia: Saunders Elsevier.

These physiologic changes are intertwined with the emotional and spiritual gifts of breathwork. Just as you exhale and inhale physically, so you also *breathe* spiritually. Throughout time, breath has always been considered inextricably linked to health, consciousness, and spirit. In ancient Greek, *psyche pneuma* means breath/soul/air/spirit. In Latin, *anima spiritus* translates to breath/soul. In Japanese, *ki* is air/spirit; and in Sanskrit, prana connotes a resonant life force. In my practice of Christianity, breath is often described as the indwelling of Spirit.

Breath control is the gateway to self-regulation, returning us to present moment awareness. By balancing the breath, we synchronize our body systems and settle into an alert but calm state. By harmonizing the body systems, it creates an internal environment conducive to opening up to grace, peace, perseverance, and the many spiritual muscles that are needed for resilience and personal transformation.

Below, I break down some simple "steps" for you to work through with the breath. As you practice, these steps will become a seamless experience and a natural part of your breath awareness.

1. Approaching a Mindful Pause for formal practice, you assume a comfortable seated posture and become aware of your breath. Notice how it might inform you of your current state of being. Is it shallow? Rapid? Are you holding your breath? Turning your attention to the breath allows you to re-inhabit the body. We can easily become disconnected from the body when habituated to lead with thinking, paying less attention to feeling.

2. After meeting yourself in the moment, you can begin to settle into a comfortable pace and rhythm, lengthening the range of motion of breath slowly … smoothing out any jerks or pauses.

3. Slowly, bring balance to your breath, perhaps counting four or five counts to the in-breath and balancing with four or five counts to the out-breath. Settle into a comfortable pace and

rhythm … maintaining balance in the breath … feeling balance and stability in the body.

4. With the balanced rhythm of your breath as your guide, you can begin to scan the body, looking for hidden pockets of tension, fatigue, or discomfort. Breathe in peace and stability; breathe out tension, fatigue, and distraction. You can do this systematically, moving head to toe, or you can let your intuition or self-knowledge guide you. In chapter two, you reflected on your personal stress warning signals. Check in with your "teachers." They communicate how you "wear" or experience stress in your body. You may visit these areas first to recharge and restore areas where you know you need it most.

5. As you bring each part into awareness, you have no other intention than to sustain your balanced breathing as if your breath is moving in, around, and through that body part. By your focus on the breath, you invite the possibility for the body to respond to the "letting go" of each out-breath—letting go of held tension, fatigue, or discomfort in any form.

Studies show that when we focus on a particular body part, we effect exponentially more change in that area than if we are distracted. We see the application of this in strength training. A trainer working with a client on a bicep curl can get significantly more work out of the bicep if the client's focus is there and not chatting about plans for the weekend. Anchored attention on each body part with a quality of peace and stability trains the mind, body, and spirit for sustaining this awareness.

You can spend two minutes at this step of the practice or twenty or more. As you come to know your physical Personal Stress Warning Signals, you may simply want to visit those body parts for self-care.

Think

The Think step invites you to practice the concept of detachment, which is a common theme in meditative traditions and is described in numerous ways in the Buddhist, Hindu, Jewish, and Christian traditions. Detachment involves loosening our grasp on the world, the people, and things that reinforce our fundamental orientation toward possessiveness, control, and judgment of self, others, and situations— all of which can lead to suffering.

Mindset of Anchored Attention. Moving into the Think part of the practice, *sustain anchored attention on the breath and awareness of the body.*

- Simply notice when distracting thoughts or sensations come into your awareness and let them pass without judgment, expectation, rejection, or attachment. This "emptying" brings a sense of peace and lightness of being as you "unload" tension, judgment, and attachment.

A successful sit is one where you accept yourself and each moment as it comes along. You want to sustain peace with what is and let go of judgment, expectation, control, denial, or any other attachment. Distractions come in many forms—a thought, memory, insight, or physical sensation. Thoughts can be pleasant or unpleasant.

One thousand times, your mind may be pulled out of the present moment … and one thousand and one times, you gently return to your grounded and wakeful presence.

For most of my clients, learning to work with the fluctuations of the mind is the most relevant for supporting change and personal transformation. You may find that you are anxious, distracted, sad, or angry and label it an unsuccessful practice. If you return attention to the next breath within the chaos of thought or the disturbance of the body, it is practice. There does not need to be a good or bad. It just is.

With gentle compassion, you simply allow ... release ... and return. You notice, and let go. Meditation meets you where you are with no judgment or expectation, just perfect peace where compassion for self can grow. It is difficult to extend peace and compassion into the world if we don't know it and practice it within.

Some distractions may be pleasant, like a memory of a special time with a loved one. Or you may experience insight into a problem that you've been stewing over. While it may be tempting to savor these experiences, they interrupt your ability to remain unmoved in focused attention. By habit, our minds freely follow preferences, plans for the future, or events of the past, and seek out or even manufacture problems. In formal practice, we train to let go of even the pleasant experiences for a stretch of time. You can decide how long. This trains your discipline for focused attention. Focused attention is a valuable skill for work performance and interpersonal relations.

Thoughts are not bad. They just don't fit the purpose of formal practice, which is to sustain present moment awareness. Other times, you may use the Mindful Pause intentionally to generate positive emotion from a memory or other inspiration to expand thinking for creativity or problem-solving. But in formal practice, the "Think" step sustains a narrow focus to build the muscle of detached awareness.

Formal practice is dose responsive. Even two minutes can strengthen your attention and improve self-regulation. The clients I see making the most significant progress have integrated formal practice into their self-care routine on a regular basis. This is the step that affirms that you are not your thoughts, which brings many practitioners profound peace.

Where are you? Really? When my oldest daughter was about three years old, we went to visit her grandparents. Upon arriving at Grandma and Grandpa's house, we asked her, "Where are you,

Meredith?" She looked a little confused; and pointing to herself, she replied, "Right here."

Asking yourself where you are sounds silly. But you might be surprised to realize just how often you aren't where you think you are. This is why formal practice is so important. It's quite amazing how you can feel steady in your practice, completely present, and all of a sudden you find your mind has drifted back to your office rehashing an incident that caused you to be upset or drafting the grocery list you need for the week! How did you get there?! How long have you been there?!

Even these questions are part of the distraction … another problem to solve. But your meditation time is not for solving problems. This is why it is called the monkey mind. The mind can be tricky in pulling your attention away from your focus. Simply practice noticing when you've left the present moment, and with the next out-breath, release the thought and return to the breath and sensation of peace in your body.

How are you being present? The goal is being present with peace and compassion. Probably the most difficult thing is to be aware of the essence or quality of the relationship with your mind in doing this. When you notice distraction, are you frustrated? Disappointed? Angry that you're not "successful"? Emotional hooks are common triggers for distraction, and as previously discussed, they have the potential to alter our physiology into an incoherent state. Maintaining peace with breath regulation and body awareness stabilizes our emotions and maintains physiologic harmony. This is the real "work out" phase of your practice. Anchored in peace, free of distractions, we practice self-compassion to grow our capacity for extending compassion to others.

Dealing with Resistance. Wisdom to support your practice can show up in the most unlikely places. A metaphor that I find useful for my practice came out of a kayaking experience along the shore of Lake Superior. I was there to explore the sea caves up close. I was out with a guide who was explaining why they have to be mindful of the size of the waves. A two-foot wave is the limit for safe kayaking due to a concept known as "rebound." When a two-foot wave comes in from the big lake and hits the cave wall—a resistance—that resistance amplifies the wave, and it rebounds off the cave wall as a two-and-a-half- or three-foot wave. This can make kayaking challenging at the least, but possibly dangerous for novice kayakers.

The phenomena of "rebound" is similar to what happens in the mind when we put up our own "wall of resistance" to thoughts or emotions that we don't like or are trying to avoid. Notice in the guidance above to release and let go. We don't stop, block, or push away our thoughts. This resistance only amplifies the thought—making it more difficult to sit with a clear and steady mind. If we approach our practice with the intention to notice resistance in body or mind and meet it with a quality of peace and stability, we find that like an uninterrupted wave, a thought may come, rise in its intensity, and then pass. Staying tethered to our breath as an anchor and the sensation of peace in the body helps us ride out the waves of distraction that will inevitably show up in our practice.

There are some common "waves" that you can count on to use as practice. Physical sensations are great teachers. It's not uncommon while in sitting meditation to have an itch capture your attention, maybe on your leg ... or on your nose. It's a strong, trained habit to react to the sensation without thinking. Use this as practice for "allowing." The sensation to react will appear. Notice it. It will grow in intensity like a wave ... and sometimes, it will pass without a need to respond to it by scratching. Give it a try. Set a timer for a 5-minute sit. Anchor your attention on the breath and the sensation of peace in the body. Your ability to notice ... allow ... and then choose if, when, and how to respond is a resilience skill that helps you navigate distractions through the course of a day that can knock you off course.

The attention you strengthen in formal practice will help you apply the skill in your "informal practice." You can also use a common trigger like your phone ringing or pager going off. When you are interrupted, stop, breathe, and think of anything that shifts you to inner peace and stability before choosing if/when/how to react.

The varied guidance for meditation requires dedicated practice and often requires the help of a teacher, guide, or coach. You can find teaching aids through books, workshops, retreats, online, or in person. You may want to do a little research to determine what style or approach best suits you.

I offer a basic four-week mindfulness challenge on my website. Each week is dedicated to an element of the Mindful Pause. Daily emails contain an inspirational image, quote, and tip to grow your practice. Periodically, I offer retreats to practice these skills, unplugged from life, and plugged into moment-to-moment awareness in a beautiful setting. Clients experience profound shifts, just beginning with the simplicity of the Mindful Pause for meditation.

Choose

We have to empty ourselves to be filled up.

–Mother Teresa

The steps of stop, breathe, and think hold a quality of "emptying" that frees us from the burdens of body, mind, and spirit and opens space to be filled up. What will fill this space? Positive emotions and energy.

A connection to our heart is one of the best ways to generate and communicate positive energy to the mind and body. We can use the gift of spaciousness that we created when stopping, breathing, and freeing the mind, to fill ourselves intentionally with the positive emotions that have the power to uplift, energize, and change the way we see ourselves and the world.

This last step, "choose," transitions our beingness back into our doingness with the upward spiral of energy that we generate from a strong connection to our heart. Connecting to your heart broadens your awareness beyond the breath and builds the energy to choose how you want to move out of your practice and into the world to live into your life of deliberate actions … not simply reactions.

3 P's of Positivity. There are a number of ways that you can generate a strong heart connection. As you begin to broaden your awareness beyond the breath, allow your imagination to create a scene that generates a swell of positive emotion. I find that there are **3 P's of Positivity** that work well for most people:

- Person – someone you love or care for deeply
- Place – somewhere you feel safe, serene, or inspired
- Pet – need I say more? Often, just the suggestion of a pet brings a smile to many faces.

Take your time to bring your target into clear focus. Be very detailed in your visualization, engaging all five senses if possible. Allow your visualization to move beyond just the thought of your target to an actual felt sensation of being in that scene. Having been anchored in your body for your practice, you will likely notice the shift in energy that you feel in your body when you generate an authentic experience of your scene. Your mind doesn't distinguish between what's real and what is imagined. I suspect this is why post-traumatic stress disorder is so difficult to heal. But just as the brain has the capacity to "relive" traumatic experiences, it also has the capacity to be moved in a positive direction by intentionally recalling our most powerful positive moments.

Shift Mindset to Expand and Grow. It's important for me to highlight here that as you transition into the heart connection, you are *shifting from a narrow focus mind to one that taps the power of expanded awareness and growing energy.* As your ability to visualize fuels your body, mind, and spirit with positive intention, you may sense the growing energy as anticipation, enthusiasm, eagerness, drive, or passion.

Additional "heart connection" options could be turning to your devotional reading, practicing movement meditation like yoga, tai chi, or Qigong, or expanding your meditation to other practices that cultivate a positive emotion.

Sharon Salzburg and Pema Chodron teach a beautiful Tibetan meditation practice called Tonglen Meditation that cultivates empathy. Loving-Kindness is another Tibetan form of meditation that grows compassion. There are a number of daily devotionals inspired by a variety of sources that share wisdom and inspiration to support personal growth.

> *A multitude of beautiful options exist to connect your inner self to your outer world, creating a seamless connection between your truest self and your lived experience.*

The formal practice of a Mindful Pause is not meant to be experienced in a vacuum. Mastery comes when the "you" that sits in practice becomes the "you" that you take into the world—a "you" who is grounded, intentional, and able to recognize distractions and sustain peace.

Just the beginning. The Choose step marks the end of your meditation practice. But it is truly designed to be the *beginning* of a state of being that prepares you to move with steadiness and optimism through the complex interactions of your day. This is why most meditative traditions practice in the early morning, before the start of a day. Your Mindful Pause practice, like the rise of the early morning sun, gracefully wakes up the body and mind and wraps up with the warmth, energy, and inspiration of a new day. Sometimes, it's tempting to have your "Choose" practice BE your practice. It's a little like eating dessert first! And I sometimes do that! But I make it a deliberate and intentional choice.

> *I continue to find that when I meditate in the morning before work, I have a better outlook on the day and a better day in general.*
>
> –Coaching Client

You can find an audio guide of a five-minute Mindful Pause on my website: www.guidedresilience.com.

It can be valuable to reflect on your Mindful Pause experience. Consider journaling after your practice. Some questions you might ask include:

What did you notice? What were you aware of? What was present? What showed up? How might the Mindful Pause impact how you show up in the world? Or how you react in different situations? How might this skill help you stay well? Or reduce stress?

Take a moment now to consider how you would like to experiment with a Mindful Pause meditation practice. Where will you practice? For how long? How will you remember to practice?

Chapter 8

Mindful Pause for In-the-Moment Mindfulness

Do you ever find yourself:

- ☐ Rushing through activities without being attentive to them?
- ☐ Breaking or spilling things because of carelessness, inattention, or thinking of something else?
- ☐ Failing to notice subtle feelings of physical tension or discomfort?
- ☐ Lashing out at a friend, colleague, or loved one without thinking?
- ☐ Preoccupied with thoughts of the future or the past?
- ☐ Snacking without being aware of eating?

Mindful Pause, in the moment, provides a means of sustaining mindfulness in the "doingness" of our lives. I usually introduce this skill early in the coaching process with clients. It provides immediate relief and support. In fact, for many of my clients, they refer to the tool as their Rescue Pause. It has the ability to protect against having a moment stolen by the distraction or harm of depleting emotions. The Mindful Pause, then, when integrated into our day, guides a more informal practice to grow our mindfulness skill, lead more intentional lives, and deepen our appreciation of all moments of life.

Mindful Pause, in the course of daily living, is a quick remedy to come back to yourself. Randomly checking in with yourself, you will likely find that you are not in the present moment. And when you catch up with yourself, you might discover the quality of your awareness is far from peace. It is so easy for the mind to slip off into the future or slink back into a past event.

Have you ever driven a familiar route and arrived at your destination not able to recall the details of your commute? Perhaps you drafted an important email in your mind, completed a grocery list, or rehashed a conversation with your spouse … but you weren't fully present to your drive. Driving, especially a familiar route, tempts the brain to do what it does well, which is moving conditioned patterns of behavior to a more unconscious regulation. This wouldn't be so bad if not for the fact that on any given day, there are a multitude of uncontrollable factors that play into a commute—the weather, other drivers, road conditions, or pedestrians. So the commute can be a great informal Mindful Pause practice opportunity that improves your safety by keeping your hands and your attention at the wheel.

So, let's break down the Mindful Pause practice—Stop … Breathe … Think … and Choose … for **in-the-moment regulation.**

STOP

When do you stop? When you notice one of your stress warning signals. That is why self-awareness is such a critical resilience skill.

Wellness coaching is a valuable engagement to grow this skill. For example, I had a phone session with a new client who had not yet been introduced to the Mindful Pause tool. She works as a nurse and had recently moved into a new role. She's highly trained, driven, experienced, and a perfectionist. She had recently been diagnosed with a disease that made the physical toll of her day difficult to manage.

In her new role, she noticed there were situations, tasks, or questions from patients or their families that were new and unfamiliar to her. She was accustomed to the confidence that comes with experience. Subsequently, she found herself "bumbling over her words," "feeling like an idiot," and "unable to think clearly." Not only was she enduring the uncomfortable sensations that accompany a new role, but she added to her suffering by beating herself up with harsh criticism. She was able to describe clearly her personal stress warning signals. Having a sense of where this was going, I prepared to share with her the Mindful Pause tool.

Together, we examined the situations that caused her to be upset and what being upset or uncomfortable felt like for her. How did she know she was upset? Exploring the situation more deeply, she was able to identify some triggers and the values or motivations behind her behaviors (exploring the "equally true").

I then asked her what remedy might alter her reaction to future situations. She was silent for several seconds. When she spoke, she said with a sense of ease and simplicity, "I think I just need to pause." I then shared the Mindful Pause tool … and she chuckled. She had worked her way to this very powerful remedy by examining her situation and tuning in to her own intuition—very satisfying for both of us. What would your stressful situations feel like if you were able to recognize the need and take a mindful pause in the moment?

BREATHE

*Life is in the breath. The one who
half breathes, half lives.*

−Chinese Proverb

Breath as Teacher. The next step, breathe, is essential. Awareness of your breath may be one of the signals that precipitates the use of a Mindful Pause. The breath is a great teacher and indicator of your mood and energy. Our breath can become jagged when we are angry or upset. We may hold our breath when concentrating intensely on a project or task. Or we might gasp out of fear or grief. The breath is inexorably linked to our emotions. So with breath control, we gain access to a powerful ally in self-regulation, self-discipline, and emotional control. The breath begins the shift to peace in body, mind, and spirit that facilitates the power of the pause.

Most people move through their day with little attention to the breath. We relegate the breath to our unconscious mind and expect that no conscious awareness is necessary. While it is a great relief that we don't have to direct our body to take every breath consciously, we miss a lot of valuable feedback when we don't cultivate an awareness and control of our breath. We grow this relationship in the formal practice so that our awareness is heightened in lived experience.

Breath helps you re-inhabit the body. The breath is tactile. It has a physical sensation that brings you back to your body in the present moment. Too often, we are disconnected from our bodies, relying heavily on the information processing of the brain to direct our actions. But the body has critical information that informs our choices. Even a single, intentional, full-range-of-motion breath can bring you into the present moment … or a state of mindfulness.

Breath brings you to the present moment. The present moment is a powerful vantage point. Often, our stress response is heightened when our mind travels back to the past or into an imagined future. Both the past and the future have a role in our experience of living well, but too often, those thoughts hold emotional triggers that derail our composure and critical thinking.

Even a single breath creates a gap of sorts between the present moment and your reaction to it. In the gap, you regain your power … your sense of autonomy … your self-control. Autonomy is a key element of well-being and resilience, and we are at our best when we are intentional and deliberate in our actions. From this present-moment perspective, you are able to tackle the third step, Think.

THINK

Direct Experience – Right Mind. Having already connected to your body with the breath, the "Think" step quickly recalls the stability and peace that you memorized in your formal practice.

Consider the quality of your moment-to-moment experiences. Attend to the direct experience of each moment, absent of the commentary that often misdirects attention (and energy) away from what's real. This observer mind is a practice of detached awareness, free of judgment, expectation, or attachment to a particular outcome. The ability to observe from this stance grows in formal practice. It interrupts the storytelling that takes up space in our mind. Releasing the distraction of commentary, imagining, supposing, or analyzing requires awareness and practice. The following are common distractions that, with awareness, you can remedy rather quickly.

Control/No Control

One of the first things to consider when experiencing stress is whether the trigger is within your control to change or not. Escalating emotions over things outside our control is wasted energy. Rehashing these events over and over in our minds feeds that energy drain.

Stealing From the Present Moment

In yoga, there is a teaching around "non-stealing." Many assume this means taking material property away from another. But it also suggests considering how many of us are likely to be tempted to steal from our own peace of mind in the present moment. This happens every time we lose ourselves to worry or rumination over things that are not real. Consumed by past events and future outcomes can be a needless drain of energy over what is not real in the present moment.

Sometimes worry can be worthwhile. If worry prompts you to be vigilant and take action to be prepared, safe, and alert, then it has served a higher purpose for self and likely others. Once the proper safeguards are in place, you can let the worry go. It no longer serves a purpose, and it only steals from your enjoyment of the present moment. It is no longer the "right action" for the time. There are no hard and fast rules about the appropriate amount of worry. This is yours to discern mindfully in each situation. Your body, mind, and spirit will communicate with you, sending you signals that inform how you can best show up in certain situations.

Highest Good for Self/Others

Self-care is a holistic journey toward living with intention into your meaning and purpose. Happiness is not the only objective. Happiness has more to do with having needs satisfied, getting what you want, and feeling good. Meaning is more related to uniquely human activities, such as developing a personal identity, living into your intentions, and consciously integrating one's past, present, and future experiences.

Clarity around your life's meaning, purpose, and your unique strengths and core values is needed to give you confidence that you are living in alignment with your personal mission. Meaning reflects one's identity but also transcends narrow self-interests. This balance guides you to the highest good for self and others.

A Mindful Pause deepens self-reflection and guides to right action. It's helpful to ask the question, "What thought or action would serve the highest good for others and myself?" This usually reorients you to the wisdom inherent in a strong connection to your core values. It empowers you to be a person of deliberate and thoughtful action who does not simply react to situations. Reactions are often inspired by our selfish nature. Using the Mindful Pause generates the coherence that connects us to our higher brain functions of empathy, compassion, and kindness to consider the right action. It helps to do the following mindfully:

- Choose words when interacting with spouses, children, or colleagues.
- Curb anxiety when starting a new job or task or participating in certain social situations.
- Regulate emotions during a commute.

The Mindful Pause disarms the thoughts and sensations that lead to unbecoming behaviors. Some are surprised how quickly initial tendencies (e.g., impatience, judgment, or expectation) fade when making an effort to stop and take a grounding breath to interrupt the reactions that usually follow certain triggers. For example, commuting often holds the potential to derail any peace that you may have generated in your morning practice of a Mindful Pause. I experience interesting insights when I practice the Mindful Pause on my commute. Part of me is competitive. As a runner and basketball player, I was trained to navigate around competitors or aggressively guard my space in pursuit of a goal. It may be the "right action" in some circumstances, like competition, but it isn't the best quality of awareness to tap during my morning commute. My meditation and mindfulness practice grow my awareness of the variety of motivations that exist. When I use my Mindful Pause to recognize the presence of my competitive self, I give space for the peaceful self that I cultivated in my morning practice to show up and preserve the commute as a continuation of steadiness in my core, resistant to the emotional hook of my competitive side.

A Mindful Pause conserves personal energy. Self-care is never selfish. Experiencing just enough positive return on these initial "experiments" is a minimal investment that often inspires continued personal practice because you quickly experience the value of preserving your energy so that it can be better spent sharing with those you love.

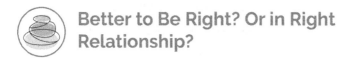 ## Better to Be Right? Or in Right Relationship?

Mindful Pause preserves relationships. Often, our first impulse (being "right") is a natural, but selfish, thought. It's all about me. The Mindful Pause allows space for that very natural tendency to be balanced by a deeper discernment that considers both personal commitments or desires AND the needs of others.

What is the "right action" or "right relationship"? That is a very personal determination that comes out of alignment with your beliefs, values, and personal strengths. In addition to alignment with self, right action and relationships align with your social environment and societal commitments. Mindfulness maintains that alignment as we engage in our very complex and challenging lives. Your "right action" options appear as you connect to renewing emotions.

CHOOSE

Choice is a powerful tool. The Mindful Pause guides you to a choice point where you can "Choose" right action. Even in the face of events that are definitely outside of your control, you can retain a sense of personal power with a Mindful Pause that gives you space to transform how you respond to those events. It empowers you to become a person of deliberate action, not just reaction.

A day can feel overwhelming when filled with a constant barrage of interruptions that sometimes provoke thoughtless responses either out of habit or as a result of the pace and intensity of our day. The Mindful Pause puts the brakes on this "out of control" sensation and empowers you with choice and focus. And that provides relief.

Choose to interrupt multitasking. The Mindful Pause can also help you navigate the tendency to multitask. No matter how mindful we are, we cannot change the reality that competing commitments will continue to fill our days. With a Mindful Pause, you can put your attention on one task at a time. Easing the weight of your day one moment at a time can make the difference between a day where you struggle to maintain 50 spinning plates in the air, to one that builds in ease and purposeful intention one plate at a time, moment by moment, ending the day in the win column.

This practice protects against fracturing your attention or holding awareness of an unbearable load. This possibility comes as a great relief to many who feel overwhelmed at the end of their overly full days. It doesn't mean that you move through life in a state of bliss or a tortoise pace. A Mindful Pause simply gives you space to catch up with yourself and restore coherence, ensuring informed and deliberate choices for the highest good for self and others.

Choose to wake up to the miracle of every moment. The impact of the Mindful Pause came to me with a smile when I sat down to write this chapter. There is a quote by Paulo Coelho from his book, *The Alchemist,* that says, "And, when you want something, all the universe conspires in helping you to achieve it."[20] My family was vacationing, and I was committed to writing a couple of hours each day. I intended to write about the gift of present moment awareness that comes with a Mindful Pause. I didn't want to miss out on an entire day with family, so as they headed out for an excursion, I stopped and connected to my breath. Thinking of my core values, I chose to trust that I would find a spot to write as they explored.

We ended up at an arboretum. My Mindful Pause presence let me see with possibility. I ended up seated on the ground with my laptop at the edge of a fountain that had the most beautiful lotus flower blooming. The diversity of tropical colors was enchanting. Dragonflies zipped by. A breeze interrupted the intensity of the sun. Birds were singing. I intended to write about the Mindful Pause practice, and the universe gifted me with one as I prepared to write in this beautiful setting. Sitting cross-legged at the edge of the fountain, I *stopped*. Awareness of my breath brought me fully into the present moment. My body relaxed as I settled into balanced breathing. My mind became alert and focused, and my heart was awed by the scenery around me. I woke up to the wonder of the present moment.

Many practitioners of meditation and mindfulness describe a sense of "waking up." I've read this from great spiritual masters and heard it from clients who are experiencing mindfulness practices for the first time in their life. For me, *this* is the most profound and beneficial aspect of growing a personal mindfulness practice, and it is what keeps me returning to both formal and informal practice for more growth. The fruit of waking up can be harvested whether you're a novice or expert meditator.

---

[20]   Coelho, Paulo. *The Alchemist.* 2014. New York: HarperOne.

The Gift and Challenge of the Present Moment

The Gift of Present Moment Awareness

When my oldest daughter, Meredith, was about six years old, we shared a very special Mindful Pause. We had a hibiscus tree that we kept in our dining area, just off the kitchen. One morning, we woke to find that one of the plant's buds had opened into a beautiful flower. We celebrated this "opening up" with the excitement of expectant parents. We studied the flower deeply, examining the color, the shape of the petals, and the interesting stigma, stamens, and anthers. It was fascinating. Later, when my husband Steve was at the breakfast table reading the newspaper, Meredith excitedly encouraged her dad to "look at the flower!" He was deep into whatever he was reading and didn't respond. She encouraged him again, "Daddy, look at the pretty flower!" Steve, holding his paper in front of him, turned to look over his shoulder toward the hibiscus and then returned his gaze to his paper. Maybe there was an utterance of acknowledgement … I don't remember. What I do recall is what Meredith said next. She said to Steve, "Daddy, when you looked at that, did you see *something*, or did you see *nothing*?"

As you move throughout your day, it is easy enough in any moment to stop, check in with your breath, and fully inhabit your body. Breathing in stability and peace, you can then check in with your thoughts and savor the present moment. This savoring allows you to choose to connect compassionately to the reality or "somethingness" within every moment. A Mindful Pause is a gift to yourself that will reward you with insight, inspiration, and right action.

The four simple steps of the Mindful Pause have been transformative for many of my clients. I give clients a magnet that they often post as a visual reminder to interrupt the stress response or to savor the "somethingness" of each moment. They'll often ask for a couple, as they find it helpful in a variety of places. They'll post it at their work station, in their car, at home on the fridge, or in their bathroom to view at the start of a day. These four simple steps can improve relations in the workplace, encounters with spouses and children, personal reactivity to difficult situations, and coping with anxiety and fear in the face of life-threatening health situations.

Many people describe a mindful state of being when practicing an art form or being in nature. I have experienced the deep satisfaction of mindfulness in sculpting clay on a pottery wheel, scuba-diving in the ocean, and walking with wonder and awe in a variety of places in the natural world. So many practices lend themselves to the restorative power that comes through a deep connection to self and integration of self with the world. I've had clients who work with animals, plants, or music to experience deep engagement in moments of personal satisfaction. Invite mindfulness to emerge in all the ways you live and move and engage in the world.

 ## The Challenge of Present Moment Awareness

For moments that are beautiful and inspiring, awareness is a gift. It is rewarding to savor these times. But for other moments, like the ones that provoke feelings of sadness, fear, judgment, or anxiety, many people hope that learning meditation will help them escape these emotions and just plug into bliss. That is not the purpose of mindfulness. Resilience grows when you allow mindfulness practices to connect you deeply to every moment, trusting that every moment holds an opportunity to choose to live into right action as opposed to simply reacting to the world. You can learn to accept, work with, and transform the full range of your human emotional experience.

Another client of mine refers to the Mindful Pause as her Rescue Pause. She says, "It saved my life." And she's quite serious. I met her when her mother was dying, and her marriage of twenty-five years was unraveling. Life seemed to be tailspinning out of control. No technique can fully take away the pain of difficult life events, but the Mindful Pause and the breath, in particular, can resource you in ways that allow you to be fully present and deliberate in thought and action.

A Mindful Pause is an act of self-care that allows space for the practice of accepting what is—even when what is is not the most comfortable place.

Consider the stressful experience of losing car keys. Imagine this happening on a day when you overslept, it snowed six inches, and you have an important meeting scheduled that morning. The accompanying emotions of anxiety, worry, frustration, and anger make it very difficult to access memory because of cortical inhibition, or incoherence. You recognize your stress warning signals in a shift toward depleting emotions. You take a cleansing breath that brings you back to the present moment, letting go of worry about being late or what your colleagues will think of you. Another breath helps you release frustration and harsh criticism of yourself for not placing your keys in their designated spot!

This coming back to yourself makes space for you to think. You generate positive emotions by connecting your breath to the deep gratitude you have for your family, your work, and even the snow that you know your kids will enjoy that day. By generating coherence with the renewing emotions, access to memory returns. In addition to saving your family the upset of your charged reaction, you are able to recall that you had borrowed your husband's coat the night before to run a quick errand. You find your keys there.

Like lost keys, life affords us many opportunities to experiment with a Mindful Pause to interrupt disruptive reactions. Shifting into present moment awareness with breath regulation and a renewing emotion, you regain cortical facilitation, and your response is thoughtful and productive. Intermittently bringing yourself back to yourself in the present moment is a powerful way to practice self-regulation. You can practice this in the flow of your life and work.

> "On days where it may not be easy to meditate early, I still try to find opportunities to tap into the current of connection."
>
> –Lisa, a hospitalist and mother

Using the Mindful Pause for mindfulness can also prevent or interrupt habituated reactions that lead to poor choices. Integrating a Mindful Pause into your morning commute guards you from the distractions of traffic or rude drivers so you can remain anchored in your breath and your ability to see, hear, and touch the reality of the moment, releasing any frustration with the next out-breath.

The Mindful Pause can also ground you before a difficult meeting or conversation. It can put the brakes on automatic reactions that don't serve the highest purpose for others or yourself. Several clients have used the Mindful Pause to get through interviews or difficult performance evaluations. When you want to present your best self, the Mindful Pause elements of stop, breathe, think, and choose maintain your alignment with your best self and highest good.

I've noticed that staying grounded in Mindful Pause presence helps me "hear" better as well. Training the mind to stay present captures details in speech, body language, and other subtle cues, which makes communication more productive and satisfying. It has also greatly improved the ability to remember peoples' names. I can't tell you how many times in casual introductions my mind wanders away from the present moment, and in less than 15 seconds, I've forgotten a name. Most likely, I never heard it in the first place! I was probably distracted by planning the next question in my mind. With disciplined practice, you train your ability to recognize being pulled out of the present moment. I'm sure you can imagine all kinds of settings where present moment awareness could enhance your life.

CASE STUDY: THE MINDFUL PAUSE FOR IMPROVED PERSONAL AND PROFESSIONAL PERFORMANCE

Situation

Stephanie, a physician assistant in a busy oncology clinic, was dissatisfied with her ability to cope with the overload she was experiencing at work. This was affecting her satisfaction with work and relationships with colleagues. As a thorough and highly efficient provider, she had prioritized patient care but at a high price. Her mood and energy were depleted, and her relationships with colleagues suffered. She sought out coaching to address self-regulation. It didn't require a huge time investment for Stephanie to experience a significant shift in the perception of her work and a subsequent improvement in relationships.

Desired Outcome

- Establish and maintain a dedicated program of self-care for body, mind, and spirit.

- Become more mindful and less reactionary in stressful situations.

Stephanie's Impactful Program Elements

- Completed her MAP to identify vision, strengths, motivations, and gaps.

- Learned Personal Stress Warning Signals that lead to reactionary behavior.

- Established use of the Mindful Pause to interrupt the stress response and act mindfully.

- Observed habits of feeling irritability and overwhelm, and identified the patterns, people, and situations that trigger this habit.

- Integrated the Mindful Pause practice strategically throughout the day to regulate mood and energy.

- Developed both formal and informal mindfulness practice to support skill development with Mindful Pause.

- Engaged the CHIP model for self-reflection.

Stephanie's Results

Stephanie made a simple lifestyle change, adding the use of the Mindful Pause to regulate mood and energy throughout her hectic days. Skilled use of the Mindful Pause, along with mindfulness practices, resulted in her recognizing her "cues" and then having the ability to adjust to those cues, which made work life easier and more pleasant. She also noted that these changes filtered into her personal life as well, and she experienced more contentment and happiness overall.

Enter the Laboratory of You

Consider a situation or two that come to mind which might benefit from a Mindful Pause:

1. Record the situation.

2. Note your stress warning signals, or how you will know the event upsets you.

3. Describe your desired result from a Mindful Pause.

4. Have fun experimenting!

I have had clients experiment with driving in traffic, engaging with in-laws or difficult coworkers, or exploring a new social group or hobby.

One of my own fun experiments? Heading to a check-out line at the grocery store:

Stress Warning Signal: My competitive edge kicks in. I scan the store quickly, looking for my "competition." I anticipate who is attempting to beat me to the finish (or check-out lane). I grip the cart, furrow my brow, and tense my arms and shoulders. I'm ready to take out anyone who gets in my way!

Desired Result: I want to free myself from this unnecessary competition. I won't win any medal for cutting off my neighbor in a fight for "next in line"! The Mindful Pause gives me space to recognize my silly attachment and choose to let it go. This makes room for a sense of peace, not hijacked by hurry.

This may seem trivial. But when you begin to notice how much better you feel in the small, letting-go choices, you realize how, if uninterrupted, they can quickly accumulate and add to a day of stressors that drain your energy.

The Mindful Pause makes space for possibility to grow. As we progress through this work, you will learn additional nuances and skills that add to, amplify, or lead to diverse applications of this life-changing skill.

Breathe Takeaway

Mindful Pause for Self-Regulation. To live with intention into your most authentic life requires mastery of moods and energy. When you are strong in body, mind, and spirit, and trained in self-awareness, temperance, and compassion for self and others, you naturally align your thinking with your life philosophy or values, bringing you a deeper sense of meaning and purpose. The Mindful Pause tool gives you access to grow awareness and skill at self-regulation.

Think

I can't change the direction of the wind, but I can adjust my sails.

–Jimmy Dean

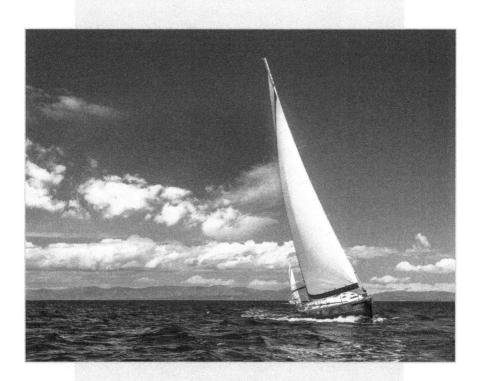

Chapter 9

The Path of
Intentional Living

Guided Resilience coaching is an approach that draws from two prominent pillars of positive psychology thought:

- Values in Action (or Strengths)
- Emotional Agility

Intentional living takes discipline and focus. For some, the very thought of discipline and focus takes on qualities of drudgery or painstaking effort. Do discipline and effort have to be hard and uncomfortable? Not always. Personal values and emotional regulation can help.

The two most impactful motivation and change strategies that can help bridge the gap between knowing and doing are an awareness of personal strengths and the ability to harness the power of positive emotions.

Strengths

Sometimes along the path of life, we lose a solid connection to our personal strengths and values. Usually, this occurs as a result of external motivations or commitments. Or perhaps we start to believe that work has to be hard to be worthwhile and productive.

One of the most meaningful outcomes of wellness coaching is remembering who you are. By knowing and using your strengths, nurturing positive practices and relationships, and learning self-regulation skills for emotional agility, life can be energizing and rewarding.

You considered your strengths when creating your MAP. As mentioned there, I also encourage clients to complete the VIA survey to help identify character strengths and values. Prior to assigning the VIA, many of my clients struggled to identify their strengths when designing their wellness vision. They simply couldn't name them. Without knowing your strengths, it's likely you'll create a wellness plan inspired by "shoulds" and not the "wants" that make your plan meaningful, enjoyable, and therefore, sustainable.

It's fascinating to see the diversity of wellness visions that people arrive at by aligning with their strengths. Your most satisfying pursuits and the best tools to support your well-being will be born out of your own connection to your deepest and truest sense of self.

Ben recognized just how important an awareness of strengths could be when navigating important life moments.

CASE STUDY: LIVING INTO YOUR STRENGTHS

Situation

Ben is a young professional, married to another professional, raising one child with hopes of growing their family and their careers while preserving a strong connection to other dimensions of well-being.

Desired Outcome

Learn self-regulation skills to navigate the complexity of sustaining current life commitments and living into a desired life with confidence and intention.

Ben's Important Program Elements

As part of onboarding, Ben completed the VIA Survey of Character Strengths. At our first meeting, he was able to articulate a compelling life vision (MAP) that expressed his desire for career advancement that would give him financial security and personal satisfaction applying his growing professional skills.

Results

Within a couple of weeks of boldly expressing his intentions, he was approached by a former employer inviting him to return. As it turns out, the new job would satisfy most of the hopes that Ben had articulated in his vision.

The job opportunity was a bit overwhelming to consider and triggered some significant stress warning signals that were quite uncomfortable. It's not uncommon in stressful situations to hone in on the problem at hand and the uncomfortable sensations of dread, anxiety, and confusion that often accompany them.

By the time of our next session, Ben described the events that transpired around his new job offer. These included surprising accommodations that were made to recruit him and having a difficult conversation with his current employer. Though quite stressful, Ben had made it through a very challenging and exciting stretch. Remember the roller coaster reference? Ben was on quite a ride! We were both amazed by the timing of this new opportunity and how it aligned with the vision he had crafted only a week or so before.

When Ben shared his story of how this all unfolded, he revealed a connection to his strengths. Ben's top five character strengths are: Judgment, Fairness, Creativity, Honesty, and Gratitude. These virtues showed up all through his story.

He used his judgment to discern what he had to have in order to make a change in employment. His fairness made him mindful of the impact of his decision on his current employer. A strong lure to the new job was the opportunity to use his creativity to craft the new job design. Ben was honest with himself, the recruiting company, and his current employer.

Ben further aligned with his strengths by expressing gratitude to his current employer for the valuable work experience as well as to his new employer for the serendipitous job offer. Ben felt reassured recalling the "blessing" of his family when he recognized the presence of his stress warning signals. This eased the intensity of the stress that is inevitable in these situations.

When we made those connections during his session, I could hear Ben's sense of relief and reassurance. A "strength-lens" of his story had been previously unacknowledged due to his preoccupation with the insecurities that were also present in making a life transition. Focusing on the "Equally True" gave a perspective of the experience that was affirming and energizing. It's easy in challenging situations to be preoccupied with insecurity and doubt. Both can be equally true … but mindfully choosing to direct attention toward an affirming mindset generates that momentum for positive change.

> No emotion should be avoided or ignored. Our full capacity for a wide range of emotions is what makes us uniquely human. Recognizing, honoring, and mindfully navigating our emotions is the goal of self-regulation.

The impact of training a strength-lens is powerful. Intentionally living a life in alignment with strengths/values makes moments and days more satisfying and meaningful. Strengths are present even in the more uncomfortable situations as well. This challenges clients to examine what benefit, skill, grace, or strength showed up or grew out of a personal struggle or conflict (exploring the "Equally True").

Trusting that growth is possible in all our lived experiences is a powerful approach to living. And knowing and using strengths grows happiness, confidence, and resilience. Ultimately, it contributes to overall well-being.

The Power of Positive Emotions

Love is a better teacher than duty.

–Einstein

Emotions are energy. They can energize and uplift, or keep you calm and relaxed. They can agitate, and they can drain. Awareness of your emotional landscape is a resilience skill that grows out of Mindful Pause living. With peace as your anchor in the Mindful Pause, you become witness to the fascinating and complex nature of your emotional experiences.

With respect to positive emotions, Barbara Fredrickson led the way with investigations into several positive emotions.[21] She determined that even brief touches of positivity can begin to alter how you view the world.

Why is positivity important? Positivity is important primarily because it feels good, and you are more likely to choose and repeat behaviors in a positive mindset. When pursuing lifestyle changes, it helps to connect your desired actions with your strengths and values. When you experience this alignment, it generates positive emotions that ensure consistent implementation of new behaviors.

Emotional Shifters. Barbara Fredrickson studied ten different positive emotions, including joy, gratitude, serenity, interest, hope, pride, amusement, inspiration, awe, and love. She described how positive emotions could broaden thinking and build resources that support personal growth. Her work is supported by evidence showing that coherence—the physiologic result of authentic positive emotion—facilitates cognitive function and fuels resilience.[22] Her research further details that cultivating positive emotions is a learnable skill that contributes to human strength, resilience, happiness, and ultimately, well-being.

Positivity does not ignore suffering or difficult emotions. Difficult moments still interrupt intentions for a good day. In fact, being indifferent to your own depleting emotions may affect the way you are present to others. Being dismissive of suffering or glossing over situations with inappropriate positivity may communicate an unwillingness to empathize with another's pain by giving them the impression that you lack care or concern for their situation.

---

[21] Fredrickson, Barbara. 2009. *Positivity.* New York: Crown Publishers.

[22] Rozman, Deborah, and Rollin McCraty. 2013. "HeartMath." *www.heartmath.com.* https://store.heartmath.com/item/2075/emwave-solution-for-better-sleep-guide.

What would be appropriate positivity in the presence of pain? Simply your peaceful presence to what is. You don't have to take on the heartbreak of others to show compassion. Anchoring yourself in peace and choosing the supportive energy of love and kindness are what give you the confidence and courage to show up in situations that need authentic care and presence.

Cancer survivors know the disappointment of separation when those around them lack the confidence to regulate their emotions. Many describe the friends that "disappeared" during their personal crisis. It takes courage to be present for those who are suffering. Living into the Mindful Pause gives you a practice to lean on. You learn to grow the stability of peace and courage so that you choose faith, hope, and love. These feelings nurture both you and the wounded you encounter.

Emotions, both positive and negative, are contagious. Emotions have the power to either pull others down with you or lift them up. Warriors for authentic care and peace can interrupt a downward spiral with an infusion of kindness or humor that redirects the emotional traffic. Managing moods can be difficult, especially if you work in an environment where people unnecessarily create drama or in professions like healthcare or social services where emotional challenges are a constant presence.

Negative emotions are sticky. Negative emotions are regarded as "sticky," like Velcro. We tend to remember situations, people, and events that cause upset. While this may be helpful in some situations, it is not always worth the energy cost and cognitive inhibition that accompanies the depleting negative emotions.

Positive emotions tend to slide away quickly, like something on Teflon. Evidence of this is recognizable in the common exchange of, "How are you today?" Often, what first comes to mind are frustrations, like being stuck in traffic or weather ruining plans. Work breaks can shift to sharing the latest dramas. There's nothing inherently wrong with these tendencies. But if self-regulation is a goal, then awareness of the nature of interactions and how they impact your mood can direct choices.

Tipping point for positivity. Fredrickson described a target ratio for tipping mood in favor of the positive. Evidence shows that a ratio above 3-to-1 forecasts flourishing. What this means is that for every negative emotion, you need three positive emotions to return to an energetically renewing state. This doesn't sound so difficult until you consider a typical morning routine—rushing to get kids off to school, yourself ready for work, traffic, and the news! For some, it is routine to start a day in the hole.

It is predicted that 80 percent of Americans fall short of the 3-to-1 ratio that predicts flourishing. And this ratio is for "normal" conditions. Environments laden with strife (i.e., a difficult marriage, poor work culture, or sick family member) can bump the ratio up to 5:1 or even 10:1. Sounds like more opportunities for self-regulation and the Mindful Pause.

Likely, you will be experiencing stress warning signals that alert you when your emotional energy has shifted. With this information, you practice your Mindful Pause. There is so much power in the pause. You can collect yourself, breathe, be mindful of anchoring in peace, and choose to infuse the next moment with one of many appropriate renewing emotions.

 What's your ratio? Fredrickson's website has a brief inventory with only 20 questions used to calculate your positivity ratio. You can find it at PositivityRatio. com/Single.php

Emotional Agility

Emotions are energy, and mastering emotional agility is a resilience skill. Emotions can empower or sabotage personal growth. Interestingly, both positive and negative emotions can generate an energy that supports the right action. Anger can make us creative, selfishness can make us brave, and guilt is a powerful motivator to reconcile differences. The book, *The Upside of Your Dark Side*, explores the fascinating impact that a variety of typically negative emotions can have on behavior.[23]

Emotional agility follows a Mindful Pause that allows you to return to the present moment with a calming breath. It creates a gap where you can recognize your current state so you can consider whether your emotion is generating the appropriate energy to support the best intentions for yourself and others. With awareness, you experience the autonomy to choose your right action.

I have a client who works as a receptionist in a cancer care clinic. In crafting her wellness vision, she recognized her strengths of empathy and kindness. She experiences meaningful connections with patients and is dedicated to offering support and encouragement when they visit the hospital. She welcomes patients every day who are facing their greatest fears and enduring physical suffering.

She, herself, struggles with emotional regulation. Her mood can sometimes lead to behaviors that disrupt her relationships with colleagues. Recently, she came to her session obviously disturbed. Her posture was slumped. Her expression, defeated. She described a frustration that she had experienced in her work that day. She had been offended by the action and comment of a colleague. The event consumed her.

---

[23] Kashdan, Todd, and Robert Biswas-Diener. 2015. *The Upside of Your Dark Side*. Plum Books.

She described feeling upset by the (perceived) accusation that she was not meeting the needs of the patients when reminded to keep the coffee pot full. This challenged her value of being empathetic and showing kindness to others. She regards her attentiveness to patients as one of her greatest strengths. By her retelling of the story, it was not only the actual event but the story she was telling herself about the event that generated all kinds of bleak interpretations of her situation—most of which were not real, just imagined. Her assumptions were causing her distress and draining her energy.

To help her remedy the discomfort that accompanies negativity, we experimented with the upward spiral of positivity that comes with recalling positive events in her day that were equally true. Science is now showing that gratitude is a very powerful emotion that supports mood and energy regulation. We practiced a brief Mindful Pause. She stopped her accelerated negativity to come into present moment awareness. She breathed away tension and attachment to her story. She welcomed an inner quality of peace.

I guided her to choose to reflect on any blessings that occurred during her day. She was able to recall that one of the cancer patients brought her produce from their garden as an expression of gratitude for her care and attention as a receptionist. By just retelling this story, her posture lifted, and a smile returned to her face.

What a beautiful gesture by that patient! And how affirming of her strength of caring for others. But it was lost, largely due to her inability to recognize and reverse the negativity that trapped her in a downward spiral. She discovered the "Equally True" by hunting for the good stuff. It is always there.

Reversing the downward spiral to reveal the "Equally True" takes training. Neuroscience is proving that it is worth the effort. Neuroplasticity is the ability of the brain to change continuously throughout an individual's life. It is within your reach to pattern a life that habituates positivity practices just like we've conditioned our bad habits. It simply requires disciplined practice. The exercise below is one I regularly use with clients to begin to rewire the brain for positivity.

 Three Blessings Exercise: Simply reflect on and journal about three things that went well today ... and why.[24]

That's it—what went well and why. The journaling, it is suggested, should be written, not typed. Writing takes longer, so it allows more time to savor the energy created by the event. We are attempting to reprogram our nervous system so deeply savoring these events helps to override old tendencies and habits.

Evidence suggests that positivity practices actually change the way we see the world. I encountered a woman who experienced this to be true. She had been practicing the Three Blessings Exercise, or "gratitude journaling," for over a year. She attested to the influence it had on conditioning her to see goodness everywhere she went. She began to trust it. And expect it.

Sometimes our wiring for a negativity bias is so strong that it can really feel like work to recall positive events. The "wheels" of our mind may feel like they're churning slowly or may feel stuck in the mud of our clouded lens. I start every coaching session with an invitation for my client to tell an upward spiral story of a recent event that produced positive energy.

Sometimes people really struggle with this. I had a client unable to come up with a single uplifting event. Instead, we generated positive energy with a mind-body activity to shift into the mood needed for a productive coaching session. Thirty-five minutes into our session, he interrupted our dialogue to report his recollection of a positive event.

---

[24]   Seligman, Martin E. P. 2011. *Flourish.* New York: Free Press.

He seemed relieved that he had reached an inner freedom that allowed that positive memory to bubble up.

A Mindful Pause breaks the chains of negativity that feel heavy and oppressive, allowing the lightness of being that comes with anchoring and sustaining a connection to positive restorative emotions.

My Positive Day Visualization

Visualize yourself waking up to a gorgeous morning sky with brilliant shades of pink, orange, and red. Birds are chirping as you begin your morning with meditation out on your porch. You take time to enjoy a cup of coffee with your spouse before getting ready for work. Everything seems to go smoothly. Even your commute was a treat. There was a detour due to construction, but you welcomed the new route as entertaining. You noticed a small café that you'd like to try.

You catch yourself smiling as you head into work with a light and eager step, thinking of the fun you had on the weekend with friends. A colleague returns your smile with a smile and offers to assist you in getting ready for the morning meeting. Even your daunting email inbox doesn't dent your mood. You're in an upward spiral of positivity that seems to grow in strength and casts off any irritations that otherwise might trip you up.

Or consider this scene: You wake up irritated with yourself for socializing too late into the evening. Your irritation led to an argument with your partner about who was responsible for dinner that night. The start of a construction project added to your commute time and frustration as you noticed every other annoyed driver along your path. Your pace was brisk and sharp as you approached your office with a sense of dread. You avoided eye contact with your colleague to ensure that you wouldn't be delayed anymore. You rifle through stacks of folders, getting a painful papercut in your haste to prepare for the meeting that started five minutes ago. Amidst this chaos, you swear that you can hear your computer screaming at you—shaming you for not taking time on your weekend to clear your inbox.

Likely, you've experienced both kinds of days. Pleasant moments lead to pleasant days—despite frustrations and disappointment. Take it one Mindful Pause at a time.

Chapter 10

Traps, Nuggets, and Connecting the Dots

Life is a journey, not a destination.

–Ralph Waldo Emerson

These are terms I like to use when talking about life experiences that become meaningful moments. "Traps" are habits or behaviors that challenge you. They can make significant growth or change difficult.

"Nuggets" are the coaching theories or perennial wisdom that help you manage "Traps." Nuggets can give clarity to sometimes murky and confusing Traps. They can be actionable tools or mantras – or an inspiring "refrain" - to help you work through difficult situations. It can feel like a "Eureka!" moment when a nugget suddenly makes sense and then becomes part of your lived experience.

"Connecting the Dots" attempts to illustrate how the variety of Mindful Pause tools work together to manifest your best life vision.

Ultimately, your own experiences—whether victories or challenges—are your best teacher. Nuggets of wisdom, insight, or shortcuts can lighten your load, lift your spirits, untangle your confusion, or clear your lens.

You probably have some awesome nuggets of your own, and I'd love to hear about them! You can send them to me through my website: GuidedResilience.com.

 ## Trap: Fixed Mindset and Negative Self-Talk

Nuggets:

- Growth Mindset: A million ways to solve a problem.
- Reframing situations with the "Equally True."

Connecting the Dots:

- Mindful Pause to check your "Mindset."
- Negative self-talk generates incoherence and blocks creative problem-solving.
- Hunting for the "Equally True" taps the power of positive emotion, creates coherence, and results in several options.

Carol Dweck coined the terms fixed mindset and growth mindset to describe the underlying beliefs people have about their intelligence and ability.[25] A person with a fixed mindset assumes that human qualities, such as intelligence, character, and ability, are relatively stable and cannot be changed in any meaningful way. Success is the affirmation of one's inherent intelligence.

Conversely, a person with a growth mindset believes that human qualities are malleable and can be improved with effort. In this way, challenges and obstacles are viewed as a natural part of learning.

---

[25] Dweck, C. 1999. Self-theories: *Their role in motivation, personality, and development*. New York: Psychology Press.

A fixed mindset can lead one to think that there is only one right answer to a problem or situation. More often than not, there are multiple courses of action that can lead to progress. A wise teacher once shared, "There are a million ways to solve a problem." Fundamentally believing in abundance versus scarcity is a growth mindset that supports lifelong learning and growth. Why are we hesitant? Likely, because we are afraid to fail. But even falling short of our goal affords us the victory of learning, which is a valuable reward.

This reminds me of a client who was interested in growing his meditation practice. He was familiar with sitting meditation, so he intended to build this practice back into his life on a regular basis. He had studied Buddhist practices and had an idea in his mind about what his practice should look like. He came to a session disappointed that he did not meet his goal. In fact, he had not practiced sitting meditation at all. In his self-reflection, he noted his failure and called himself "lazy."

As it turns out, he had recently started a new job. We all know the increased mental and physical toll that comes with a significant change. He struggles, at times, with anxiety, so he was motivated to be mindful of his self-care during this transition. When it came to getting out of bed in the morning for formal meditation practice, he just wasn't willing (thus the judgment of lazy).

So when asked, "What did you do instead?" he explained that it wasn't that he was tired. He actually woke before his alarm but chose to use the time to reflect on the blessings in his life. He described how he found relief and groundedness in holding thoughts of his family close at the start of his day and was then able to recall the sensation during the course of his day.

As I reflected back to him what I heard, it became very clear to both of us what I was describing—*his* meditation practice! His "limited" thinking kept him locked on one version of meditation practice— formal sitting meditation. Suddenly, the energy of this situation completely changed. He could see that he **had been** disciplined in his self-care. He was meeting a need with a practice that supported his desire to remain positive and calm in a new and exciting environment.

Mindful Pause for formal meditation is intended to support your seeking, not to keep you tied to a particular practice. A growth mindset may lead you to your own restorative practice.

 ## Trap: All or None

Nuggets:

- Remember yourself.
- Do what matters to you – "do a little bit of something."
- There are a million ways to solve a problem.

Connecting the Dots:

- Be mindful of your Holistic Well-Being Circle Assessment.
- Coaching relationships support discovery dialogue.
- Use a Mindful Pause to generate a growth mindset to set SMART goals that are "Realistic."

Julian, a driven nurse pursuing her doctor of nursing practice degree, got teary during a discussion after completing her holistic well-being assessment. While her work and sleep dimensions were full and satisfying in many ways, she had neglected several of the dimensions in pursuit of her goal.

She was deeply dissatisfied with the fast food that had replaced her home cooking. And her relationship with her boyfriend was suffering due to a lack of quality time. As she described her love of cooking and spending time with friends, she smiled, remembering the life-giving energy of these activities.

Drive can be a fabulous attribute. But at what price? Further dialogue revealed options to balance out her "all or none" approach to her career. She appeared relieved and even eager to sprinkle her strenuous life with doses of "a little bit of something" that cultivates joy.

Whether you want to give something up or add a new habit or behavior into your life, it's easy to sabotage success with an unreasonable all or nothing approach.

Do you have to give up late-night TV completely to get better sleep? Or could you "try a little something" by experimenting with two nights of an alternative nighttime ritual?

If you can't run a 5K without stopping, does that mean that you should give up your gym membership and resume life as a couch potato? Or could you "try a little bit of something" by beginning a 20-minute walk/jog program two times a week?

Working with a coach, you can experience the growth potential of discovery dialogue that generates a growth mindset that leads to SMART goals.

 ## Trap: Identifying with Negative Emotions

Nuggets:

- Practice detachment.
- Recognize paradox.
- Coherence is contagious.

Connecting the Dots:

- Mindful Pause practice for mindfulness.

It is easy to fall into the trap of identifying with emotions that limit our options. We say, "I am anxious," or "I am sad." Mindfulness helps us recognize that we are not our emotions. With detached awareness, we witness, "I am experiencing anxiety." Or, "I am feeling sadness." Detached awareness allows for the possibility that emotions will pass. We don't cling to the story. Identification with an emotion can make it difficult to let go or to view a situation from multiple perspectives or a growth mindset.

What's helpful to keep in mind is the paradox that two opposing things can be true at the same time. I can feel anxious about my future AND feel comforted by the love and support of family. I can experience sadness when dealing with a loss AND allow the kindness of others and the beauty in the world to be a buoy that holds me up.

When my mother was dying, it was easy for me to be consumed by the sadness of her impending death. But I will never forget the scene of my two daughters and two of my nieces sitting at her bedside, gently singing, retelling family stories, and painting her fingernails. My body and mind felt laden with grief, but the energy of the room was lifted up by their tenderness, care, and love.

Paradox is real, and coherence is contagious!

A Mindful Pause to stop, breathe, and think about the presence of many realities in any particular moment (the Equally True) allows you to choose the lens that opens your heart to the highest good for others and yourself.

Learning to appreciate the spaciousness that comes with the "detachment" that mindfulness describes is a transformational skill. The observer mind is able to remain steady in an infinite source of equanimity and peace. Detachment is not meant to disengage, which can lead to a guarded or indifferent heart. It's meant to provide space and awareness where it's possible to embrace the paradox. The terrain of this personal path of awareness becomes familiar with practice.

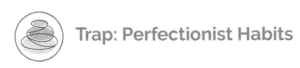 Trap: Perfectionist Habits

Nugget:

Progress not Perfection

Connecting the Dots:

- Practice trial and correction.
- Recognize hidden commitments.
- Engage in coaching and/or the CHIP self-reflection tool to grow self-awareness. (This will be explored more in the "Choose" section).

In addition to an abundance mindset, growth potential expands when you embrace mistakes. When pursuing behavior change, there can be a strong attachment to doing something "correctly" the first time. Experiments may be rejected if they don't go exactly as planned. This can be a very disruptive tendency. High achievers who are not accustomed to anything but excelling in their pursuits miss out on the growth potential that lives in mistakes.

Keep in mind the mantra "trial and correction" to replace the commonly held "trial and error." "Trial and correction" supports a growth-promoting lens of experimenting with change. A growth-supporting lens allows progress to replace perfection.

Inevitably, clients will cancel a session if they "didn't get their homework done." Yet, these can be some of the most productive sessions. By exploring what you DID do, you are often able to uncover hidden commitments that drive your behavior.

Hidden commitments are actions you take to defend a value, belief, or vulnerability that is stronger than the desire for change.

No matter how clear and well planned a goal may be, hidden commitments can dominate decision-making, so to root them out is a victory. Additionally, you'll uncover a deeper understanding of yourself and what motivates you that you can add to your arsenal of positive actions. A coaching relationship or thorough self-reflection with the CHIP tool can further support this growth. More to come on this option in the "Choose" section.

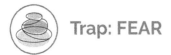 ## Trap: FEAR

Nugget:

False. Evidence. Appearing. Real.

Connecting the Dots:

- Use Mindful Pause for self-regulation.

Anxiety and worry are a common threat to well-being and happiness. I use the acronym above to remind clients of the power of the Mindful Pause to bring you into the present moment where you can observe your **direct experience. Indirect experience** can go wildly out of control, imagining all kinds of false evidence about worst-case scenarios, stories that build drama with hyperbole, and inaccurate assumptions about what others believe, did, or said. It's shocking to consider how much energy is wasted perseverating over what is not real or true.

The Mindful Pause can help discriminate between direct and indirect experiences. It helps you let go of ruminating false thoughts and surrender to the present and real moment where you can generate and sustain peace.

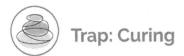 **Trap: Curing**

Nugget:

Healing

Connecting the Dots:

- Holism

One of the nuggets I learned in my professional life is the holistic notion of healing versus curing. For a number of years, I worked as a program director and wellness coach for a small nonprofit holistic wellness resource center. Our programming focused on providing integrative or complementary support for people with chronic illness—predominantly cancer.

I was initially concerned about working in this arena. I had chosen wellness and optimal performance for a reason. I feared that working with those living with or dying from cancer would be depressing and futile. Remember that F.E.A.R. is false evidence appearing real. I found my experience to be exactly the opposite.

When life is interrupted by a critical illness, some people seize the opportunity to wake up to life, their purpose, and their relationships. They see life as precious, their choices as critical, and the role of self-care as essential to their holistic well-being. I witnessed incredible courage, profound insight, and a letting go of expectations in cancer survivors that opened up possibilities for their thriving even in the midst of great suffering. I was often struck, recognizing that cancer survivors could be more "whole" than the many "presumably well" who moved through life hurried and unaware.

Those living with chronic disease were living testimony to the possibility that holistic healing is possible even when curing is not. Cure implies finality—or a destination. Healing suggests a process—a journey. Much of the pursuit of wellness involves embracing the reality of a moving target. Nothing stays the same. Trusting in this constant change is an essential part of effective coaching. It's important to know that this is an integral part of discovering authentic wellness.

The Mindful Pause process acts as a gentle reminder and guide to accept yourself as you are—no matter your current state of health or illness. We are perfectly designed in our imperfections. Healing is always achievable.

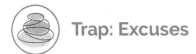 **Trap: Excuses**

Nugget:

Explanation

Connecting the Dots:

- Use a Mindful Pause.
- Pause for self-reflection.
- Anchor in strengths.

Excuses are what tend to surface quickly. The dictionary defines an excuse as a "defense, justification, and an alibi." In contrast, an explanation is a "clarification, account, and enlightenment." Regularly practicing self-reflection illuminates your vulnerability to making excuses and gives you the opportunity to be honest with yourself and take responsibility.

You can begin to recognize triggers for excuse-making with a Mindful Pause, and think, "Am I excusing my behavior or explaining myself?" That pause may give you the space to appreciate the strengths, values, or commitments that motivated your action. Self-regulating your emotions helps to communicate clearly and kindly.

 ## Trap: Attachment to Being Right

Nugget:

Is it better to be right? Or in the right relationship?

Connecting the Dots:

- Practice Mindful Pause in the moment.

Chrissy is a recent nurse graduate. She is very dedicated to her profession and recently secured a job on the cardiac floor of a hospital. She pursued coaching proactively, knowing she would be challenged personally and professionally. In reflecting on her victories for the week, she described taking a Mindful Pause in the course of conversation with her mom.

Chrissy explained, "I chose not to respond with a snarky one-off when talking to my mother on the phone, which I believe allowed her to get a little deeper into what she was talking about because she felt heard." Focusing on her relationship with her mother and listening supported her mother's need to feel heard. Her mother called back a couple of hours later, teary, thanking Chrissy for her compassionate presence. Chrissy's choice to protect the relationship was very satisfying for both.

Think Takeaway

- Know Your Strengths.
- Train Emotional Agility.
- Work with your own inner wisdom to recognize Traps, explore Nuggets, and Connect the Dots.

Choose

*In the long run, we shape our lives,
and we shape ourselves. The process
never ends until we die. And the choices
we make are ultimately our
own responsibility.*

–Eleanor Roosevelt

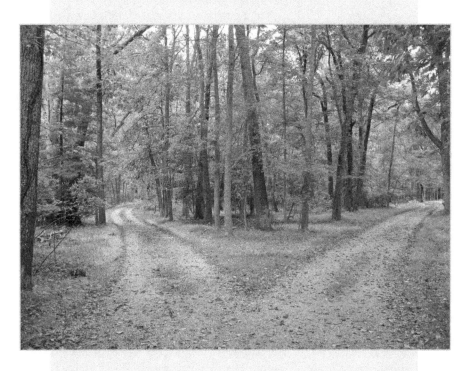

Chapter 11

Choose the Guided Resilience Path

I founded Guided Resilience so that I could live fully into my personal calling to contribute to the well-being of others. Optimal health and well-being are fully realized when you feel in control of your life and choices. Personal peace is your prize when you uncover your calling to engage in the world and contribute to the fullness of life and service to others in a way that uses your gifts and protects resources … including you!

Mindful Pause captures key elements of the Guided Resilience work I do with individuals and groups. The first section of this book started out describing the tenacious pace and intensity of life today. While not an unworthy pursuit, there are consequences to how we prioritize our time and energy. A result of this numbing pursuit is the potential to lose track of your deeper sense of meaning and purpose, which requires a body, mind, and spirit integration. The Stop, Breathe, Think, and Choose method of my Guided Resilience work invites you to grow mindful awareness of yourself and how you experience and discern your true nature, personal calling, or sacred Self.

Mindful Pause introduces my Guided Resilience approach that is grounded in evidence-based science but sprinkled with wisdom from world religions, writers, and philosophers. This combination is meant to ignite your own inner spark. Your seeking can take you on your own rich path of self-discovery. You get to *choose* how you live, move, and have your being in the world.

It has been my hope to provide the structure that allows you the personal freedom to explore your own version of transformation. In this section, I share practices from my personal and professional toolbox. These practices come from the Christian tradition, yogic training, Qigong, modern science, and the natural world.

 # Sabbath as the First Mindful Pause

I grew up in a thriving Catholic family in central Iowa. The idea of a Mindful Pause was formed in me early on since we attended church as a family every Sunday. This Sunday "pause" put the brakes on the regular routine and pace of life to gather as a community, slow down, and engage in the pursuit of wisdom, virtue, and purpose. My Christian formation inspired compassion for those who struggle with life's complexities and a desire to support the well-being of others.

Sunday worship just began this ritual of rest. The extended family would continue our Sabbath gathered at my maternal grandmother's house for a day of play, relaxation, and a great homemade meal. Prioritization of relationships was evident. Familial love was the training ground for living the intention to love your neighbor as thyself. My parents worked hard in service to others through their vocations, the community, and their church. This was also my earliest experience of the value of rest to support vitality. These were unstructured days that afforded us time with family, naps, play, and leisurely eating.

My childhood experience also embodied a core virtue explored in Mindful Pause—discipline. Fortunately for me, this discipline was a joy, not an avoidance of judgment. It was inspired by gratitude, not guilt. Without knowing it at the time, my faith formation was my first experience of the growth potential described in positive psychology. So many tenets of my Christian formation are now being actively researched through scientific studies. Love, kindness, empathy, compassion, and gratitude are just a few of the targets for a deeper understanding of how these virtues contribute to our health and well-being. And Christianity isn't the only source of this wisdom. All the great wisdom traditions and religions exist to help us discover our true Self and our true relationship to the sacred. This discovery is the ultimate peace, profound joy, and most satisfying goal of well-being.

 Take a moment to make a list of those activities that you engage in during the week that instruct, guide, model, or evoke any of these virtues:

- Love – grown and nurtured first within yourself, so you can share generously with others.
- Gratitude – a powerful "inner" antidote to the downward spiral of emotions.
- Kindness – a powerful "outward" antidote to the downward spiral of emotions.
- Peace – sustaining a calm mind and body.
- Service – living ethically, feeling good by doing good.
- Forgiveness – a mountain to climb within before extending to others.
- Grace – recognizing the sacredness in all things, in every moment.

How much time do you spend engaged in nourishing these virtues? What impact does your Sabbath presence or absence have on your life?

Choosing to live a more mindful, meaningful, and virtuous life is an exciting and powerful adventure. The steps within this book give you the evidence-based guidance that supports behavior change. It is my hope that you will experience the profound impact of keeping a holy Sabbath, or rest, as part of your wellness plan. Clients who create their sacred space and pursue a deeper understanding through the personal exploration of wisdom teachings make significant strides in their sense of mastery over stress and clarity around life satisfaction and purpose.

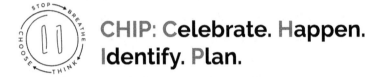

CHIP: Celebrate. Happen. Identify. Plan.

Self-reflection is often lost in the hurried pace and resulting fatigue that accompanies many modern lifestyles. The **CHIP Model for Self-Reflection** helps you grow this necessary skill. CHIP is intentionally designed to help train a particular approach for reflection. Clients are invited to reflect on a series of prompts a day or so ahead of their coaching session to bring forward key insights and connections that inevitably guide them to their authentically inspired next steps.

You can't solve a problem with the
same mind that created it.

–Einstein

It's important that the CHIP Model is approached as a mindfulness practice … not just a task or "homework" to be completed for your coach. It is designed to grow personal awareness that leads to insight. Insight and wisdom are often overlooked by sheer lack of intention. Life is too full. Commitments are too pressing. The inner work of reflection is sacrificed to the outer work of fulfilling obligations. Toward this end, self-reflection should be practiced at an unhurried pace, preferably in your sacred space or another relaxed and inspiring setting.

The "C" of the CHIP model stands for Celebration. Reflection begins with what went well with action steps. This overrides the very natural and often conditioned tendency toward negativity bias. It also produces positive emotions that generate creativity and improve problem-solving capacities.

The "H" or "Happen" prompt looks for a deeper consideration of how victories occurred. Savoring the experience thoroughly, recalling the people, environment, timing, resources, or strengths that contributed to success takes practice. As the neuroscientist Donald Hebb describes, this training trusts that the "neurons that fire together, wire together." In other words, the more time you give to training your brain to take in the good, the more it becomes a wired way of being.

After a thorough reflection of victories, your inner landscape is prepared for "I"—to "Identify" unmet action steps. This is never very difficult. The challenging part will be to recognize the strengths, values, commitments, or learning victories that are hidden in our missteps.

Judgment interrupts growth. Insight leads to positive adaptation or resilience. When you don't meet intended goals, you DID do *something*. What did you do? This often reveals hidden commitments. By recognizing these, you can make incredible advancement in self-knowledge and personal development. Honest reflection and curiosity about motivations and aversions naturally guide you to "P," the "Plan" step that seems to appear naturally.

This simple formula: Celebrate, Happen, Identify, and Plan is succinct enough not to be too time-consuming. It works with the energetic impact of emotions on thought and the motivation that naturally grows out of applying a strength-based lens to change and grow. Engaging with a coach around this process develops trust that growth comes both with success and struggle. Progress, not perfection, is the goal. Self-knowledge is the victory.

You can find the CHIP Model for Self-Reflection on the resources page of my website—GuidedResilience.com.

 # Mindful Pause Living

Regulating energy is a significant driver for pursuing change. People are just tired of being tired. Strategically integrating a Mindful Pause throughout your day helps you manage mood and energy. Making choices that align with your strengths and values contributes to a sense of autonomy that leads to flourishing. Consider scheduling a Mindful Pause at these points in your day:

- **Morning Practice** – Powerful time to set intention and mood for the day.

- **Midday Check-In** – Important not to get behind in self-care. Just like doctors recommend "staying ahead of the pain" when healing from an injury, guard your mood and energy with good choices.

- **End of Workday** – It is good practice to establish boundaries with work, and the Mindful Pause can help. Develop a creative ritual that helps you embody the choice to redirect your focus and attention.

- **Sleep Hygiene** – The Mindful Pause can be used to downregulate for deep relaxation and to clear the mind to experience restorative sleep.

For a resource guide to Mindful Pause Living with suggested affirmations to support your practice, visit the resources page of my website—GuidedResilience.com.

 # Sleep

Sleep disruption is a stress warning signal that needs to be addressed early in wellness work. When lacking sleep, there simply isn't the energy mentally or physically to make progress on positive behavior change. Here are some ways to improve sleep patterns:

1. Manage your energy throughout the day so that you aren't playing "catch up" (Mindful Pause Living).

2. Limit caffeine.

3. Move your body for at least 30 minutes—outside, if possible.

4. Limit your screen time, avoiding it altogether before sleep.

5. Establish a sleep hygiene ritual that you practice as regularly as possible.

6. Relax your body, mind, and spirit with options from this section.

 # Ta-Da! List

More than a few clients have described how their "to do" list is a source of overwhelm and dread. When it comes to work, the list is often never done. Time and energy are spent prioritizing so that important commitments are not lost in the endless stream of appointments, projects, and social activities.

The Ta-Da! List puts a positivity lens on how you view your day. Instead of feeling overwhelmed by what didn't get done or what was done late or wrong, take some time to review your day and revisit all that you accomplished. Sometimes checking items off your list is satisfying, but it can be even more powerful to write out a separate list that brings to mind …

- tasks/goals you've accomplished
- how you used a strength
- something new that was learned
- times you engaged with people in a meaningful way

Often, this list connects you into the "I want" motivations instead of being stuck in the world of "I have to's." Reflecting on your day, consider what made you feel deeply moved, engaged, inspired, or proud. Let this exercise help strengthen the being-ness of your day … not just the doing-ness.

 # Media Fast

A 2017 Stress in America Report describes that Americans care about staying informed:

> "…with most (95 percent) saying they follow the news regularly and 82 percent saying they check the news at least once each day. For nearly one in 10 Americans (9 percent), a news check-in at least every hour is the norm, and one in five Americans (20 percent) say they check their social media constantly, a significant increase from the 17 percent in 2016 who reported such use. For many Americans, news consumption has a downside. More than half of those surveyed (56 percent) say that while they want to stay informed about the news, doing so causes them stress. Further, many Americans (72 percent) say the media blows things out of proportion."[26]

---

[26] American Psychological Association. 2017. "Stress in America: The State of Our Nation." November 1. Accessed June 30, 2019. www.stressinamerica.org.

When clients are going through an emotionally challenging time, a Media Fast offers a reprieve. Emotional stress is especially fatiguing for the body and mind. Eliminating emotional upset where possible may be an important self-care practice for a time of healing and restoration.

Keep the 3-to-1 positivity ratio in mind as you lead a mindful life. If work was particularly challenging, you might prefer time in nature or with friends or loved ones instead of watching the nightly news. Knowing your Stress Warning Signals will help inform your self-care choices. I don't want to suggest that disengagement from current events is preferable. But unfortunately, "what bleeds, leads," and networks keep you engaged with emotional hooks. If you're emotionally spent, you can apply your possibility thinking and remember that there are a million ways to solve a problem. Entertainment options that generate an upward spiral of positivity are endless.

 # Think Outside ... No Box Needed

The art of medicine consists of amusing the patient while nature cures the disease.

–Voltaire

Consider tapping the restorative power of the natural world. I occasionally invite clients outside for sessions and to participate in my extended retreats in beautiful natural settings to support our wellness work. They easily sense the energy shift that nature inspires.

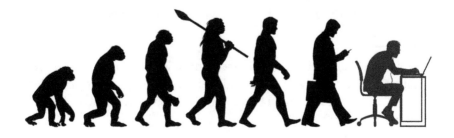

Nature deficit disorder is a legitimate concern. And perhaps it's not by accident that burnout is rampant as our time in nature declines. Research continues to provide evidence of all the ways that nature heals. One study researched nature's role in ergonomics (work setting) and demonstrated that time in nature is known to improve mood, enhance respiratory functioning, regulate hormonal malfunctions, and impact thought structure. With burnout on the rise, exposure to nature is a worthy target to consider.

How much time do you need to spend outside? A recent study examined associations between recreational nature contact in the last seven days and self-reported health and well-being. The likelihood of reporting good health or high well-being becomes significantly greater when individuals have greater than 120 minutes of nature contact in the past week. It did not matter how that 120 minutes of contact was achieved in the week (e.g., one long visit versus several shorter visits in a week).[27]

Use a Mindful Pause to consider how you might be able to tap the power of nature for restoration and healing.

Transform Interruptions Into Invitation

Interruptions are a part of our everyday experience. When cruising along with a task, a person or phone call or even our pet can intrude on our flow and fracture our attention. You might be tempted to hold one thought in your mind AND attend to the disruption. This multitasking is not only ineffective, but it is also fatiguing. Sustaining

---

[27] White, M.P., and others. 2019. "Spending at least 120 minutes a week in nature is associated with good health and wellbeing." *Scientific Reports.* June 13. Accessed August 11, 2019. https://www.nature.com/articles/s41598-019-44097-3.

present moment awareness on one task at a time enriches the quality of each experience and preserves your energy.

For this exercise, determine one or two common interruptions and a period of time, perhaps a day or week, during which you will practice transforming the interruption into an invitation to return to yourself with a Mindful Pause. The Mindful Pause will put you in a self-care gap that allows you to Choose to transform irritation into peace. If you decide that your phone will be your mindful alarm, each time it rings, tweets, or vibrates, you can ground yourself with a Mindful Pause to return to present moment awareness. I found it helpful to put the message "Smile" on my phone's home screen with an image of a beautiful flower. Then, when frustrated by interruption, I'm reminded by my screen to Stop, Breathe, Think, and Choose to smile.

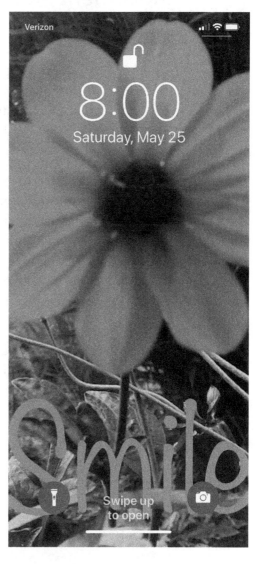

Mother Theresa said, "The smile is the beginning of peace." And there is evidence that the posture of the smile releases endorphins that improve mood. So fake it 'til you make it!

Movement Meditation

I call my body work "Movement Meditation." I incorporate yoga postures, Qigong, and good old American calisthenics! Movement Meditation is not solely a workout. By moving, breathing, and being in the body with present moment awareness, we can grow physical, mental, and spiritual strength and flexibility.

Postures have meaning. When we sit, we are receptive. We stand to deliver a speech or creed. We kneel to embody humility. We raise arms in celebration and embrace to communicate care. Brief body practices during the course of your day with an accompanying affirmation or intention help you to re-inhabit your body, connect to your source, and inspire right thought and right action. Even a mindful walk can serve this purpose. Add in a few simple stretches with positive intentions, and you have a valuable self-care practice!

You can find guides for a variety of my Movement Meditations on the resources page of my website—GuidedResilience. What we embody in our practice is intended to be carried out in the ways we live, move, and have our being in the world.

Chapter 12

Support from Others

Many Americans understand that emotional support can be crucial when dealing with stress in their lives. Nearly three in four Americans (74 percent) feel they have someone they can rely on for emotional support. That is an increase of eight percentage points since the survey first included the question in 2014. More than half of Americans (56 percent) still feel they could have used more support during the previous year.[28]

I have found it helpful in my own life to have a variety of sources for support. When my Mindful Pause reveals to me that I need a kick in the pants, I go to my brother. He's always direct and firm. I trust his counsel will keep my best interests in mind and be firmly grounded in the "highest good."

When I need compassion, I go to my sister. She is skilled at affirming my experience, which is sometimes needed before I can execute the right action. When I need something fixed, I go to my husband, Steve. He's skilled at helping me peel away my emotional sticking points to see an issue more simply. And then there's my standard poodle, Rollie.

---

[28]   American Psychological Association. 2017. "Stress in America: The State of Our Nation." November 1. Accessed June 30, 2019. www.stressinamerica.org.

When a Mindful Pause feels beyond my capacity to find peace, I find it with him.

I lost both of my parents to dementia at too young an age. Their deterioration was one of my most difficult life experiences. One evening, I was feeling particularly overwhelmed by the anxiety, sadness, and lack of control that accompanied this journey. I recognized my accelerating stress warning signals and decided I needed some time alone. I went to my room to lie down and practice a Mindful Pause. I couldn't get my breath to smooth out. My emotions had a Niagara Falls presence that was about to overwhelm me. Just when I thought I'd be swept away by a flood of tears, Rollie came and laid right next to me. His long body was adjoining mine. He couldn't be closer. He placed his head gently over my heart. He just stayed there while his coherence rescued mine.

Pets and the natural world are organically coherent. They don't experience cortical inhibition to detour away from present moment peace. Besides Rollie, I find peace at my favorite spots in nature. Lake Superior, trees, birds, the sun, the stars, and butterflies are some of my best friends. They reveal wisdom and beauty in ways that inspire the equally true. Their beauty buffers anxiety. The wonder they inspire heals wounds.

My point? Have a team for support and know how best to use them. Mindful Pause work can help you discern this important self-care strategy. Working with a coach can be a valuable asset to managing your internal and external resources of support. Coaches listen objectively. They are trained to reflect your communication back to you to reveal your strengths, hopes, and desires.

A coach works with you to cocreate your best life vision. And they keep you accountable. Living into new lifestyle behaviors may sound simple, but it is not always easy. Consider inviting a coach to support your vision, guide you to alignment with your best self, and lighten your load as you tackle expected and unexpected challenges. This is what the Institute of Coaching reported on the coaching field:

> The coaching research literature, including more meta-analyses more recently, shows overall that coaching can produce a wide range of positive effects for clients including improved self-efficacy, self-regulation, job performance, well-being, coping, and attitudes.[29]

As I finished up writing this book, I received this communication from a client I had coached more than two decades ago:

> Cami. I just wanted to reach out to you and say thank you. It was 20 years ago tomorrow that I became a runner, thanks to you. I asked you to help me get into shape (I was 244 pounds), and you said, "Great, we will put together a running program." I responded by saying, "You don't understand. I am not a runner." You looked me in the eye and said, "You are now." From that humble beginning, I have covered tens of thousands of miles, 13 marathons, countless half marathons, shorter races, and even four ultramarathons. My deepest friendships have come through running, and I shudder to think about what my health would be had I not become a runner. So, as I am 6 months from turning 60, I just wanted to say thank you for what you did for me.

At the time, I was working as a personal trainer. As a wellness coach, I rarely tell people what to do. I always ask permission before offering expertise in wellness or resilience training skills. Coaching is client-led. You can hear, however, the very satisfying sense of accomplishment he feels from working with a coach to pursue a goal and achieve even more than he had imagined.

---

[29] Institute of Coaching. 2019. "IOC Research Dose," email blast, August 11.

What do you dream of doing or becoming?

Most of my clients would agree that the issue that brought them to coaching may have been the initial target, but they experience holistic growth in most dimensions of their well-being.

> *Start by doing what's necessary; then do what's possible; and suddenly you are doing the impossible.*
> –St. Francis of Assisi

Choose Takeaway

Stop feeling overwhelmed and uninspired.

Breathe in the vitality that comes with consistent self-care.

Think in alignment with your strengths and passions.

Choose to start living into your best life today!

Gratitude

I am deeply grateful to you, the reader, for investing your time in this book so that you can learn how to pursue self-care that supports resilience. I hope you've gained confidence in your ability to live into a meaningful and satisfying life. By pursuing peace within, you contribute peace to the world. Thank you.

To my family, I owe a big debt of thanks. They celebrated the day my nine-foot table with all my notes and inspirations came out of my office, and I re-engaged in family activities. They were all patient, supportive, and so encouraging.

To my clients who share their amazing journeys with me, I give a high five! Each of your stories is a chapter in the book of wisdom held in my heart.

I have deep respect and gratitude for the field of positive psychology. It is important that a discipline promotes and protects health and wellness as diligently as we treat illness and disease.

Without the support of Niche Pressworks, I would never have completed this book. They helped me grow through the dynamic tension that shows up in taking on a personal challenge.

I'm grateful for the Source of Peace that sustains me and for the Mindful Pauses that wake me up and keep me aligned with my purpose.

Mindful Pause is a guide but also an invitation. I invite you to design the life of your dreams boldly—anchored in peace and guided by the inspirations that are uniquely you.

Peace,

Cami

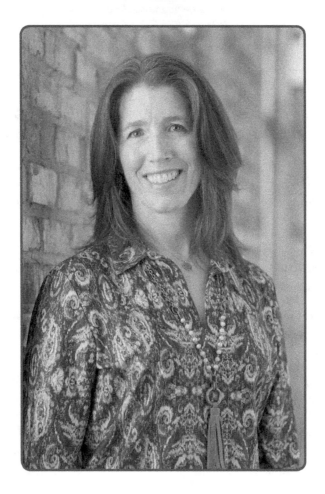

About the Author

Cami is the founder of Guided Resilience, LLC. In addition to being a professional health and wellness coach, Cami is passionate about sharing her Mindful Pause wellness strategies through workshops and retreats.

Cami walks her talk, and this book is the product of living into the Mindful Pause Process. She works from her VIA strengths which include:

1. Spirituality, a sense of purpose and faith
2. Gratitude
3. Appreciation of beauty and excellence
4. Curiosity and interest in the world
5. Capacity to love and be loved

In addition to the Mindful Pause practices in this book, she enjoys yoga, bird-watching, hiking, biking, scuba, travel, and spending time with her husband, three children, and her standard poodle, Rollie.

Cami would love to hear your nuggets, victories, questions, or suggestions: Cami@GuidedResilience.com

You can learn more about Cami and her work on her website: GuidedResilience.com

Connect with Guided Resilience on social media for inspiration and a Mindful Pause.

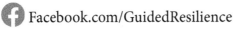 Facebook.com/GuidedResilience

@GuidedResilience

Spread peace! Share Mindful Pause with a friend.

References

American Mindfulness Research Association. 2019. *Resources.* Accessed June 30, 2019. www.goamra.org.

American Psychological Association. 2015. *Stress in America: Paying with our health.* February 4.Accessed June 30, 2019. https://www.apa.org/news/press/releases/stress/2014/stress-report.pdf.

American Psychological Association. 2017. "Stress in America: The State of Our Nation." November 1. Accessed June 30, 2019. www.stressinamerica.org.

Baard, Paul, P., Edward L. Deci, and Richard M. Ryan. 2004. "Intrinsic Need Satisfaction: A motivational basis of performance and well-being in two work settings." *Journal of Applied Social Psychology* 2045-2068.

Benson, H. 1975. *The Relaxation Response.* New York: William Morrow.

Berrigan, David, Kevin Dodd, Richard P Troiano, Susan M Krebs-Smith, and Rachel B Barbash. 2003. "Patterns of health behavior in U.S. adults." *Preventive Medicine* (Elsevier) 36 (5): 615-623.

Berutea, Beatrice. 2004. *Radical Optimism: Practical spirituality in an uncertain world.* Boulder: Sentient Publications.

Bourgeault, Cynthia. 2004. *Centering Prayer and Inner Awakening.* Lanham: Cowley Publications.

Brown, Stuart. 2010. *Play:How it Shapes the Brain, Opens the Imagination, and Invigorates the Soul*. New York: Penguin Publishing Group.

Calhoun, Lawrence G., and Richard G. Tedeschi. 2014. *Handbook of Posttraumatic Growth: Research and Practice*. New York: Psychology Press.

Chodron, Pema. 1994. *Start Where You Are*. Boston: Shambhala Publications.

Coehlo, Paulo. *The Alchemist*. 2014. New York: HarperOne.

David, Susan. 2016. *Emotional Agility: Get unstuck, embrace change, and thrive in work and life*. New York: Avery.

Davidson, Richard J., and Sharon Begley. 2013. *The Emotional Life of Your Brain: how its unique patterns affect the way you think, feel, and live-and how you can change them*. New York: Penguin Group.

Deci, Edward, L., and Richard M. Ryan. 2008. "Facilitating Optimal Motivation and Psycological Well-Being Across Life's Domains." *Canadian Psychology* 14-23.

Dweck, C. 1999. *Self-theories: Their role in motivation, personality, and development*. New York: Psychology Press.

Dyer, Kirsti A. 2002. *A Healing Place*. February 11. http://journeyofhearts.org/healing/nature.html.

Fredrickson, Barbara. 2009. *Positivity*. New York: Crown Publishers.

Institute of Coaching. 2019. "IOC Research Dose." email blast, August 11.

Jarden, Aaron. 2012. "Positive Psychologists on Positive Psychology." *International Journal of Wellbeing* 116-118.

Kabat-Zinn, Jon. 1990. *Full Catastrophe Living: using the wisdom of your body and mind to face stress, pain, and illness.* New York: Delcorte Press.

Kashdan, Todd, and Robert Biswas-Diener. 2015. *The Upside of Your Dark Side.* Plum Books.

Larkin, William. 2010. *Growing the Positive Mind.* Applied Neuroscience Press.

Lyubomirsky, Sonja. 2007. *The How of Happiness: a new approach to getting the life you want.* New York: Penguin Group.

McCraty, Rollin, and Robert, R. Rees. 2009. "The Central Role of the Heart in Generating and Sustaining Positive Emotions." In *The Oxford Handbook of Positive Psychology,* by Shane, J. and Synder, C.R. Lopez, 527-536. New York: Oxford University Press.

McEwen, Bruce, and Elizabeth Norton Lasley. 2002. *The End of Stress As We Know It.* Washington, D.C.: Joseph Henry Press.

McGonigal, Kelly. 2015. *The Upside of Stress: why stress is good for you, and how to get good at it.* New York: Penguin Random House.

McGonigal, Kelly. 2012. *The Willpower Instinct: How self-control works, why it matters, and what you can do to get more of it.* New York: Penguin Group.

Mind Tools: Essential skills for excellent career. n.d. *Burnout Self-Test.* Accessed June 30, 2019. https://www.mindtools.com/pages/article/newTCS_08.htm.

Moore, Margaret, Erika Jackson, and Bob Tschannen-Moran. 2016. *Coaching Psychology Manual.* Philadelphia: Wolters Kluwer.

Muller, Wayne. 1999. *Sabbath: Restoring the sacred rhythm of rest.* New York: Bantam Books.

Nakamura, Jeanne, and Mihaly Csikszentmihalyi. 2009. "Flow Theory and Research." In *The Oxford Handbook of Positive Psychology*, by Shane, J. Lopez and C.R. Snyder, 195-206. Oxford: Oxford University Press.

Nhat Hanh, Thich. 2007. *Living Budda, Living Christ*. New York: The Berkley Publishing Group.

Pargament, Kenneth I, and Annette Mahoney. 2009. "Spirituality: The Search for the Sacred." In *The Oxford Handbook of Positive Psychology*, by Shane J Lopez and C.R. Snyder, 611-619. New York: Oxford University Press.

Pink, Daniel. 2009. *Drive: the surprising truth about what motivates us*. New York: Penguin Group.

Rakel, David. 2007. "Integrative Medicine." In *Guided Imagery and Interactive Guided Imagery*, by MD Martin L. Rossman, 1031-1037. Philadelphia: Saunders Elsevier.

Rosenthal, Joshua. 2008. *Integrative Nutrition: Feed your hunger for health and happiness*. New York: Integrative Nutrition Publishing.

Rozman, Deborah, and Rollin McCraty. 2013. "HeartMath." *www.heartmath.com*. https://store.heartmath.com/item/2075/emwave-solution-for-better-sleep-guide.

Ryan, Thomas. 2004. *Reclaiming the Body in Christian Spirituality*. Mahwah: Paulist Press.

Seligman, Martin E. P. 2011. *Flourish*. New York: Free Press.

Siegel, Daniel J. 2010. *Mindsight:The new science of personal transformation*. New York: Bantam Books.

Smith, B.W., J. Dalen, K. Wiggins, E. Tooley, P Christopher, and J. Bernard. 2008. "The Brief Resilience Scale: Assessing the ability to bounce back." *International Journal of Behavioral Medicine* 15: 194-200.

Steger, Michael F. 2009. "Meaning in Life." In *The Oxford Handbook of Positive Psychology,* by Shane, J. Lopez and C.R. Snyder, 679-687. New York: Oxford University Press.

Walsh, Robert. 1999. *Essential Spirituality: exercises from the world's religions to cultivate kindness, love, joy, peace, vision, wisdom, and generosity.* New York: John Wiley & Sons, Inc.

White, M.P., I. Alcock, J. Grellier, B.W. Wheeler, T. Hartig, S.L. Warber, A. Bone, M.H. Depledge, and L.E. Fleming. 2019. "Spending at least 120 minutes a week in nature is associated with good health and wellbeing." *Scientific Reports.* June 13. Accessed August 11, 2019. https://www.nature.com/articles/s41598-019-44097-3.

CPSIA information can be obtained
at www.ICGtesting.com
Printed in the USA
LVHW080831151122
733169LV00026B/627

9 781946 533708